About the Author

Sarah Flower, a leading nutritionist and author of many cookery books, is passionate about healthy eating. Sarah writes for a number of publications, including the *Daily Mail*; the *Express*; *Top Santé*; *Slim, Fit & Healthy*; and *Healthista*. She appears regularly on BBC Radio Devon.

THE
PART-TIME
VEGAN

easy, delicious vegan
recipes to make
your diet healthier

SARAH FLOWER

piatkus

PIATKUS

First published in Great Britain in 2018 by Piatkus

1 3 5 7 9 10 8 6 4 2

Copyright © 2018 Sarah Flower

A CIP catalogue record for this book
is available from the British Library.

ISBN 978-0-349-42121-6

Typeset in Albertina by M Rule
Printed and bound in Great Britain by Clays Ltd, CR0 4YY

Papers used by Piatkus are from well-managed forests
and other responsible sources.

Piatkus
An imprint of
Little, Brown Book Group

Carmelite House
50 Victoria Embankment
London EC4Y 0DZ

An Hachette UK Company
www.hachette.co.uk

www.improvementzone.co.uk

This book is dedicated to my dad, who is missed every day and whose presence is felt in all my work. I think of him digging the garden when we were children, providing us with a plentiful supply of vegetables to see us through the year. At the time, I was not impressed with our small version of the good life. I used to dread finding a caterpillar in the steamed cabbage or, worse, half a caterpillar! Now, I would give anything to go back in time and thank my dad for providing my brother and me with such as wonderful, healthy start to our lives.

Contents

Introduction

We all know that our health is affected by what we eat and how we lead our lives, but it can be difficult to uncover the facts from the marketing spin and scaremongering headlines. My health journey started in my late teens when I made the decision to become a strict vegetarian, mainly because I had never really enjoyed meat, particularly fatty meats, as a child.

In my early twenties I had my first son. At 15 months old, he developed meningitis and septicaemia. It was an incredibly tough time. He managed to pull through but had some complications, so our hospital stay was extended. Keen to improve his health as quickly as possible, I asked the ward nurse if I could see a dietitian to discuss how we could improve his hospital food. She arrived carrying tins of Heinz soup! That was a life-changing moment for me, and the start of my determination to learn more about nutrition.

I trained as a nutritionist in the late 1990s, and since then my work has taken many different turns, from working with a cancer charity right through to writing books. I have been fortunate to witness some mind-blowing results from dietary changes. Our bodies are amazing, with the capacity to heal themselves when given the correct environment, ingredients and care.

I spend a lot of my time advising clients on dietary changes and ensuring that they have a balanced, nutrient-rich diet. The popularity of plant-based vegan diets has resulted in more of my clients wanting to opt for this way of eating, either on a part-time or full-time basis. As with any diet, however, interpretation is key. You can have a very poor vegan diet, in the same way that you can with any other dietary choice.

Why part-time vegan?

The definition of vegan is someone who does not eat food of animal origin. This includes dairy, eggs and honey. The diet is therefore completely plant based.

The Part-Time Vegan recognises that some people would like the benefits that a plant-based diet can give them, but still want to eat some dairy and meat; others just want to test the waters and see how they might adapt to a vegan diet. Whichever of these apply to you, this book will help you eat a balanced, real-food, plant-based diet with the focus on health. I am a nutritionist therefore I do not examine the environmental or moral argument for or against veganism, but instead concentrate on the application of a natural, plant-based diet using simple, easy-to-follow recipes that are based on everyday ingredients.

Why choose natural foods?

Today, we live in a world of convenience. Our busy lives often take priority over our food choices. Food manufacturers do all they can to convince us that their product is 'natural', 'healthy', 'low fat' or 'low sugar', and they persuade us that our grab-and-go lifestyle is healthy. Over half the food purchased by families in the UK is heavily processed, by which I mean it is pre-made so that it is ready to eat and uses mostly refined carbohydrates, chemically produced oils, fillers, additives and sugars in various forms. We have forgotten what real food is: food that is bought in its basic constituent parts – vegetables, pulses, grains, fruit, meat, fish and so on – and then home-cooked or prepared to create a meal. Have a look at some food labels and you may find that you need a degree in chemistry to decipher the ingredients list. Real food doesn't need a label.

While researching for this book, I joined some vegan forums and I was shocked by the volume of requests for highly processed food items, with most people taking the view that as long as a convenience food was vegan it was OK, or even superior. I admire the desire to avoid animal products for ethical and environmental reasons, but many people also claim that they are following this way of eating to improve their health. Relying on processed foods is, however, falling far short of a healthy diet. There is an abundance of vegan 'cheat' foods, ranging from faux meat products to faux eggs, margarines, cheese products and puddings. I understand the reasons why people might want these foods, but if you are moving to a plant-based diet for health reasons, you really need to avoid these highly manufactured foods. Any diet filled with processed food is far from healthy, and a vegan, processed diet is no exception. We are living in a society where you can be obese and yet suffer from nutritional deficiencies due to our reliance on nutritionally poor, calorie-rich, manufactured foods.

A plant-based, vegan diet can be very healthy when applied correctly. I never cease to be amazed at the difference real food can make to someone's health. Nature has given us wonderful food that is colourful, antioxidant-rich and incredibly tasty. We should celebrate this food and feed our bodies to improve our health. Yes, you do have to consider the nutrient content of your food when moving to a vegan diet, but you should be doing that regardless of the diet you follow. And if you are a full-time vegan, you will need to work a little harder to make sure you have adequate sources of omega-3 fats, vitamin B_{12}, protein, calcium, zinc and iron, but it can be done with care. Eating real food is the way to ensure your food is nutrient- and antioxidant-rich – it can also be far more economical.

The secret to a good diet, whether it is vegan, gluten-free, low carb or low fat, is always to eat food that is unprocessed and natural. I now follow a low-carb, sugar-free, grain-free way of eating. Although I was a strict vegetarian for over 25 years, I moved to a low-carb diet as part of my personal health journey. My diet remains largely plant based, but it now includes some grass-fed organic meat, oily fish and organic full-fat dairy. I listen to my body and a combination of protein-rich meat, nourishing eggs and dairy to complement a large variety of vegetables and berries is what works for me. That said, I don't eat a lot of dairy: as I approach the menopause I have found it can increase my symptoms. I have never liked milk and I drink my beverages black, but I do like yogurt, cream and milky puddings, which I often make with plant-based milk, and always sugar-free. I am flexible in my approach, but my diet is always packed with nutritious vegetables, healthy fats and good protein sources.

I love the colours and flavours of the food that nature has given us. It is far superior to the bland processed food that plays too large a part in many people's diets. This book celebrates the joy of eating plant-based foods, working with the seasons and making the most of these nutrient-rich foods.

Enjoy,

Sarah x

Part 1

THE HEALTH ESSENTIALS

Today, veganism is an incredibly popular way of eating. A diet packed with antioxidant-rich vegetables has amazing health benefits; however, if you are going to take control of your diet and aim for optimum health, you need to have a good understanding of nutrients and how they affect your health and well-being. You also need to be knowledgeable about individual food groups, such as nuts, seeds, pulses and oils – and, as a part-time vegan, meat, fish and dairy – in order to make an informed choice. There is no doubt of the benefits that including more vegetables in your diet has on your health. The grey area is how you decide on all the other factors. This part of the book provides you with a basic understanding of all the food groups and nutrients so that you can make an informed decision on the food and diet options to suit your health and lifestyle.

Chapter One

The Lowdown on Protein, Carbs and Fat

You may be familiar with the three macro nutrients that form the human diet: protein, carbohydrates and fat. Each of these plays a key role in our health, but what quantity do we really need for health? Let's look at each one in turn.

Protein

One of the main building blocks for health, protein is used for building muscle as well as other functions in the body. It is found in meat, dairy, fish, pulses (peas, beans and lentils) and some vegetables. Protein is absolutely essential for our health and we need to ensure that we have good sources of it in our diet, especially when following a vegan lifestyle.

Protein is made up of amino acids; you can think of protein as a brick wall and the amino acids as the bricks. These bricks work in varying combinations and ways to perform essential roles within our body. We have 20 amino acids, and these perform over 50,000 different functions. Nine of them are absolutely essential and are therefore called 'essential amino acids'; the remaining 11 can be manufactured by our bodies. The nine essential amino acids (histidine, isoleucine, leucine, lysine, methionine, phenylalanine, threonine, tryptophan and valine) are present in foods that are known as 'complete protein foods'. Most plant foods contain only a limited amount of protein, however, and *very rarely* in near complete form. (The exception to this is quinoa, which actually contains the complete profile.) Therefore, you have to consume much more of a variety of plant-based protein in order to reach the same volume of protein found in animal products (see the box below).

A study by the *American Journal of Clinical Nutrition* examined a variety of high-protein diets and found that plant proteins can be just as effective at building muscle as animal protein but that you do need to opt for good protein sources. Good sources of plant-based protein include nuts, seeds, especially quinoa and chia seeds, pulses (peas, beans and lentils), tofu and green leafy vegetables such as spinach and broccoli.

Vegan proteins at a glance

Plant-based foods, except for quinoa, are not complete proteins, so you need to build up a complete protein profile by combining foods. It's very simple. You can eat pulses or nuts with grains, combine pulses and nuts or add tofu or tempeh to meals. I also like to use nut butters in cooking to add a protein and flavour boost. Think about your side dishes, too, as these can give a protein boost: for example, opt for quinoa as an alternative to rice or couscous or, when making a salad, add some nuts and seeds along with healthy fats from avocado and olive or flax oil.

Carbohydrates

These are best known as our main energy source. Carbohydrates and starches convert to glucose, so a good way to think of carbohydrates is as a sugary fuel.

Carbohydrates are broken down into two forms

Complex carbohydrates are the 'real food' carbs, such as brown rice, whole-wheat pasta, wholemeal bread and so on. These carbohydrates are called 'complex' because, although all carbohydrates turn to sugar to give us energy, complex carbohydrates, which are carbohydrates in their pre-refined form, take longer to digest and release their sugars. This is because they contain more fibre and protein, which essentially slows down the digestion because your body has to work a little harder to break it all down.

Sometimes, foods that might appear to be whole-food products are actually refined, so it's important to choose your food with care (some brown breads, for example, are actually white bread with added food colouring!).

Vegetables and fruit also contain carbohydrates and therefore release sugar for the body to use as an energy source. These foods form the basis of the vegan diet, but in order to get the best nutrition from the diet without having more fuel than you need – which will result in you laying down fat – it is important to know which carbohydrates you can eat plentifully and which you should limit: for example, root vegetables have more carbohydrates than green leafy vegetables; a jacket potato is very high in carbohydrates and can contain the equivalent of up to 19 teaspoons of sugar; and berries contain less carbohydrates than other fruits such as bananas. High-carbohydrate foods also raise your blood-sugar level, which can become a serious problem leading to type-2 diabetes. For this reason, I prefer to eat high-carbohydrate foods in moderation and, in the case of vegetables, choosing to eat more of the low-carb, non-starchy vegetables.

Refined carbohydrates are carbs that have been processed, such as white flour, white pasta, cakes, biscuits, white rice and so on. In this category are also all the sugary foods that you can buy and the various different kinds of sugars: sweets, 'healthy' grain bars, cakes, biscuits (which contain sugar as well as refined flour), most chocolates, and so on.

Can we have too much?

The UK Eatwell Guide, designed by the Food Standards Agency (FSA), was put together to give a visual guide in the form of a plate divided into sections for each food type. The intention was to show people how much of each food group we should be eating in order to have a balanced, healthy diet. It currently recommends quite a large percentage of daily food to be from carbohydrates, so we assume that it must be healthy. To be honest, however, I am not a big fan of this eating guide, because it advocates a high-carbohydrate diet, which I believe is not suitable for everybody. We are told that carbohydrates are essential to health because we need them to make glucose for energy and for feeding the brain, but, unlike fats and protein, we can survive quite well without them. When you eat a low-carbohydrate diet, your energy sources come from fat and not high levels of carbohydrates. There are various levels of low-carb diets. Some people, especially those with type-2 diabetes, reduce their carbs to about 20–30g a day to make a positive change to their insulin resistance, but others eat up to about 100g per day of carbs. While it is not necessary to follow a low-carb diet if you are a vegan, as I explain later, it is worth considering reducing carbs a little, because vegan food can be very carb heavy.

As we have seen, all carbohydrates provide us with energy and convert to glucose, but refined carbohydrates convert to glucose much faster than complex carbohydrates. This is especially important information for anyone who is experiencing weight gain or who has type-2 diabetes. If you think about eating a chocolate bar or a glass of juice (which lacks the fruit fibre) – the body doesn't have to make a huge amount of effort to break those foods down. Eat a steak with some green leafy vegetables, on the other hand, and your body has to work a lot harder to digest the food, keeping your blood sugars in balance and helping you to feel fuller for longer.

How refined carbohydrates can make us fat

When we consume refined carbohydrates, we get a quick burst of glucose. This puts a process in place to help move the glucose out of our blood. To do this, the pancreas secretes the hormone insulin. This helps to push the glucose into the liver and muscle stores, where it sits in the form of glycogen, ready to be burned when needed. However, these stores are actually very small and, with our Western, higher carbohydrate diet, they tend to stay full. When these stores of glycogen are full, the excess glucose converts to fat and is pushed into our fat cells to be stored and effectively locked away. In this form it is very hard to burn, especially the fat that is found around the abdomen and vital organs, known as visceral fat.

How carbohydrates affect our feelings of hunger

A diet higher in carbohydrates also stimulates a hormone called ghrelin. Ghrelin is a greedy little fellow, who is constantly hungry, shouting at us to feed ourselves more and more. The process of stimulating insulin and ghrelin also has a knock-on effect with another hormone called leptin. The hormone leptin signals to our brain when we are full, but this can become dulled or turned off if we consume excess carbohydrates or fructose (a fruit sugar occurring naturally in fruits but which is also produced by a manufacturing process from corn and used as a sweetener in foods).

The end result is a cycle of eating lots of carbohydrates, sugars and fructose, which results in you storing more fat and craving more food. (I examine sugar and fructose in more detail later in this chapter.)

Choosing carbs wisely

Carbohydrates are in abundance in a plant-based diet, in the form of nuts, seeds, pulses, vegetables, fruit and grains. As a part-time vegan, I recommend that you choose your carbohydrates wisely. A plant-based diet is naturally quite carb-heavy, so it is important to opt for only complex carbohydrates and to try not to overload on them. Choose a diet rich in vegetables, as colourful as possible. Fruit is wonderful, but it is high in fructose, so always eat fruit in its whole from, never blended into a smoothie, where you are drinking more fruit than you would normally eat, or in a juice, which is free of fibre and so results in pure sugar flooding your liver (I elaborate more on fructose on page 34). Berries are my absolute favourite fruits as they are low in fructose and very healthy.

Whenever possible, also consume your complex carbohydrates with a little protein to help to slow down the digestion further.

Fat

We've all been brainwashed into fearing fat, but it is absolutely vital to our health and plays a key role in multiple functions in the brain, nerves, skin and joints. Fat can even help with weight management. When we talk about fat, we use different names, some of which can be very confusing. I have summarised in basic terms what each name means below, but bear with me – even touching upon the topic of fat necessitates quite a bit of detail because it is such a complex topic!

Saturated fatty acids You are probably familiar with saturated fat. It has been portrayed as the villain that contributes to heart disease. When I was growing up, at the height of the low-fat revolution, adverts showed thick globules of fat to demonstrate how our arteries would suffer if we dared to eat this bad fat. When we think of saturated fat, we visualise thick, solid fat and, to some extent, this is correct because saturated fat is solid when cold. But saturated fat is not the demon we were led to believe.

Saturated fat plays a vital role in our health and is essential for many functions, from brain health through to boosting our immune system. Furthermore, it is present in more types of food than you might have thought; in fact, all foods containing fat, contain three fats: saturated fat, polyunsaturated fat and monounsaturated fat. The ratios might surprise you as well. I recently attended a conference by Zoe Harcombe, a leading food researcher, and she shocked the audience by demonstrating that skimmed milk contains more saturated fat than unsaturated fat. Omega-3-rich mackerel contains 1.5 times more saturated fat than a sirloin steak and a tablespoon of olive oil could contain more saturated fat than a 100g pork chop. Saturated fat is found in animal products, but also some plant-based foods such as coconut oil.

You are probably also wondering about the connection between saturated fat, cholesterol and heart disease. I explain this in more detail on page 16.

Polyunsaturated fatty acids (PUFAs) are found in both plant and animal foods. These fats are found in seeds, cooking oils, some nuts (such as pine and walnuts) and oily fish. Polyunsaturated fats can contain two types of fatty acids: omega-3 and omega-6 fats.

Linoleic acid is an omega-6 fatty acid, a type of polyunsaturated fatty acid. High levels of omega-6 in the body have been shown to be very inflammatory (meaning that it can create an environment that leads to ill-health). Omega-6 fats are found in lots of highly processed oils, such as sunflower oil, corn oil and soya oil, and for this reason I recommend using oils from natural food sources, such as coconut and olive oil (preferably cold-pressed extra virgin), and avoiding all other liquid oils and margarines.

There are three types of omega-3 fatty acids: alpha linolenic acid (ALA), docosahexaenoic acid (DHA) and eicosapentaenoic acid (EPA). ALA is found in plants, such as flaxseeds, chia seeds and nuts, but it is quite hard for the body to convert it for use, especially because our diets tend to be higher in omega-6 fats, which negatively affect the process. It is generally advised, therefore, that we get our essential omega-3 fats from EPA and DHA, which are found in oily fish and some animal foods.

If you are vegan, fill up on omega-3 fats from sources such as flax oil, flaxseeds and chia seeds, but keep your consumption of omega-6 fats down in order to try to achieve a balance. This will also help your body to convert more ALA into the active forms of EPA and DHA.

Monounsaturated fatty acids (MUFAs) Monounsaturated fats are liquid at room temperature but solidify when in the fridge. The most common monounsaturated fat is called oleic acid, which is an omega-9 fatty acid found in vegetable and animal fats, but most commonly known for being in olive oil. Monounsaturated fats have been shown to help protect the heart and can improve insulin resistance (which causes type-2 diabetes and increases your risk of heart disease) and can help you to lose weight. The best monounsaturated fats include olives and olive oil, avocados, almonds, eggs, red meat, peanuts and cashew nuts.

Medium-chain fatty acids (MCFAs) Coconut oil, which I recommend in the recipes, is a saturated fat and a MCFA oil. The MCFAs make it easier to digest. Coconut oil contains lauric acid, which is also found in breast milk. It has antimicrobial properties as well as being anti-fungal. Because it is quickly absorbed by the body, it is taken up as an energy source, which means that it is less likely to become stored in the body's fat cells. It also helps us to feel full. There has been some interesting research into the effects of MCFA oil on weight, showing that it can help to keep us leaner, burning more of our stores of visceral fat (the fat around the internal organs).

Trans fats are created during the chemical process used for producing seed oils and margarines, and are found in numerous processed foods. They have been linked to heart disease and Alzheimer's and should therefore be avoided. Although the hydrogenation process that creates trans fats has changed in recent years, smaller quantities of trans fats still remain in processed foods. Trans fats can also be found naturally in dairy products and meat, but these are not the same as man-made trans fats and do not contribute to heart disease.

Triglycerides are a fat found in the food we eat and is also produced by the liver. Triglycerides are stored in the liver or fat cells but are also found travelling in our blood. High levels of triglycerides contribute to heart disease, type-2 diabetes and fatty liver disease. Alcohol consumption and some medications, such as beta-blockers, can also raise triglyceride levels.

Why do we fear fat?

Fat has been demonised since the late 1970s, but the low-fat dietary guidelines really came into force in the early 1980s. The research behind the low-fat advice is, however, fundamentally flawed. In the 1950s, a scientist, Dr Ancel Keys, undertook research into the diets of people from 22 different countries to see if the consumption of saturated fat made any difference to the rising incidence of heart disease. However, his conclusion – that eating saturated fat raises blood cholesterol, which then causes heart disease – was based on the results from just six countries because they best supported his theory. Over and above that, it was also an observational study and didn't prove that the two were causally linked. Despite these fundamental flaws, at a time of concern over rising levels of heart disease, this research was used to form the health policies for the Western world, promoting a diet low in fat and high in carbohydrates, and low-calorie diets for weight loss. We have since seen a dramatic increase in obesity and type-2 diabetes.

Despite this, the low-fat message is still championed by many and remains the basis of much mainstream health advice today. Most of my clients, for example, especially those who are overweight, have heart disease or are type-2 diabetic, have been told to avoid fat and to eat low-calorie food. Today, we have a dichotomy: we eat less fat than ever before, and yet obesity, diabetes and other conditions related to inflammation are increasing rapidly (as are cancer and Alzheimer's disease). If we listen to the latest health advice, we are getting fat because we eat too much and don't exercise enough. Did we suddenly all become greedy and lazy since the late 1970s? I think not.

We fear saturated fat, but, as mentioned earlier, it is absolutely essential for our health, from the brain, nerves and lungs through to heart and joint health. Fats also work with protein to make the cell membranes, and we need fat in order to absorb fat-soluble vitamins such as vitamins A, E, D and K. Furthermore, healthy, natural fats do not make you fat – fat keeps us feeling fuller for longer.

Although natural fats have been demonised, we've been encouraged to embrace man-made polyunsaturated fats and oils. Most of the so-called healthy fats, such as rapeseed and sunflower oils, are promoted because they are low in saturated fats; however, the processing of these oils destroys any health benefits they might originally have had. These industrially produced oils are often made using genetically modified sources and contain additional ingredients to help to give them a longer shelf life: one example is butylated hydroxyanisole, which has been shown to be carcinogenic, can lower the immune system, and can cause infertility problems and even organ damage. These oils go rancid and toxic incredibly quickly, especially when exposed to heat, light and oxygen. They cause havoc in our body, attacking our organs, our cell membranes, including our red blood cells, and even our DNA. Man-made polyunsaturated fats are also shown to increase our risk of insulin resistance and, coupled with our high-carbohydrate diet, ultimately type-2 diabetes.

We need, therefore, to opt for more natural, stable oils, such as butter, coconut oil, extra virgin olive oil or avocado oil, and to try to gain an equal balance between omega-3 and omega-6 consumption. Natural fats are very slowly starting to be valued, but, at the moment, too many people are still consuming omega-6 oils excessively and very low levels of omega-3 fatty acids. This excessive consumption of omega-6 fats causes whole body inflammation (because they are pro-inflammatory, whereas the omega-3 fats are anti-inflammatory), especially when combined with a diet of highly refined carbohydrates and sugars. You can perhaps start to understand why we are experiencing major health problems.

What about cholesterol?

Our fear of fat is based largely on the much-publicised connection between saturated fats and high cholesterol. We associate consumption of saturated fat with heart disease, yet this is now proven to be wrong. Dr Aseem Malhotra is a leading cardiologist and campaigner for healthy food. He has worked tirelessly to dispel any link between saturated fats and heart disease, proving that it is in fact our Western diet, rich in carbohydrates and sugars, that is causing our heart and our waistlines to suffer.

In fact, we get just 20 per cent of our cholesterol from the food we eat. Cholesterol is needed for almost every function in the human body, from nerve and brain function to digestion and cell health. It is present in every cell membrane, helping to maintain structure and stability, and it also helps to repair cells and tissues. Our bodies produce up to one gram of cholesterol a day to help synthesise hormones, such as oestrogen, progesterone, testosterone and cortisol. Cholesterol is also vital for brain function: 60 per cent of our brain is made up of fat and cholesterol. Cholesterol also helps us to digest fat and convert sunlight to vitamin D, which in turn helps to lower blood pressure.

What are HDL and LDL?

HDL (high-density lipoproteins) and LDL (low-density lipoproteins) are not cholesterol. They are the lipoproteins – special particles made up of fats – that carry cholesterol around the body. Lipoproteins also carry triglycerides and phospholipids.

HDL is considered to be the good kind of cholesterol transporter, as it carries cholesterol out of the cells and back to the liver to be broken down, or to the endocrine glands to be converted into hormones. LDL is considered to be the bad kind of lipoprotein because it transports cholesterol from the liver to the cells, but labelling the two kinds of lipoprotein as 'good' or 'bad' is an oversimplification because both types of lipoprotein are essential to the way the body operates and the body has ways of regulating them if there is too much of one or the other.

Low-fat guidelines claim that increased LDL levels indicate you are consuming too much saturated fats and need to opt for a better diet; however, the role of cholesterol is to provide structure and support for cell walls, so an increase in LDL might actually be due to the body trying to repair damaged cell walls.

The liver also produces more cholesterol when we are stressed or suffering from ill health and inflammation. LDL particles can be large or small, and it is the small, oxidised particles that appear to be linked to inflammation and ill health. Oxidised small LDL particles are also the result of the effects of harmful free radicals – which cause damage to cells, proteins and DNA (see box below). A diet rich in antioxidants such as blueberries, pecan nuts and walnuts, however, as well one that avoids processed foods (particularly those containing trans fats), is one of the best ways to keep your heart healthy. In fact, a diet rich in carbohydrates would seem to be the cause of a higher incidence of harmful small LDL particles, coupled with an increase in triglycerides.

Antioxidants and free radicals explained

Antioxidants are substances found in food, and naturally in the body, that can protect the body from oxidation, a chemical reaction that produces free radicals (unstable molecules in the body that can lead to premature ageing, cancers, heart disease and cognitive degeneration). Free radicals can be formed in the body or come from an external source such as pollutants, cigarette smoke, toxins, poor diet and even stress. A diet rich in antioxidants, such as vitamin C and E, can help keep free radicals under control. Foods that have high levels of antioxidants include berries (especially blueberries, goji berries, cranberries and blackberries), pecan nuts, artichokes, red onion, tomatoes and even very dark chocolate. However, most natural foods contain some form of antioxidant so try to eat a diet of real food with plenty of colour. And don't forget herbs and spices – they contain plenty of antioxidants, so fill up on turmeric, cinnamon, ginger, chilli, oregano and parsley.

The subject of cholesterol is a complex one with many twists and turns; for example, a recent study published in the *BMJ Open Journal* found that 92 per cent of elderly people with high cholesterol levels lived longer. *The Great Cholesterol Con* by Dr Malcolm Kendrick, makes fascinating reading and references many studies showing that reducing your cholesterol level might, in fact, increase your risk of cardiovascular disease. I also recommend looking at the work of Dr Aseem Malhotra, a leading UK cardiologist. There are other factors to consider when looking into the causes of heart disease, such as the role of triglycerides, the negative role of our consumption of inflammatory man-made oils, vitamin D deficiency and other factors such as smoking and stress, all of which can cause damage to the arterial walls, increasing the likelihood of blood clots forming.

Balance your fats

Technically, you can obtain omega-3 fats from a vegan diet by consuming nuts, seeds and flax oils; however, as explained earlier, this plant form of omega-3 is not readily converted by the body, especially if your diet is rich in omega-6 fats and oils. It is therefore important to avoid processed oils and margarines. If you are a part-time vegan, opt for fat in its natural state as found in oily fish, butter, meat and eggs, and, if fully vegan, eat plenty of nuts, seeds, coconut oil, olive oil, flax oil and avocados.

If you are deficient in essential fatty acids, your body will soon let you know. You might suffer with poor wound healing, dry skin, brittle hair and nails, poor concentration, depression and joint pains, which could all be down to a lack of good, healthy fats.

Chapter 2

Getting Your Nutrient Balance Right

We hear a lot about a vegan diet being deficient in certain nutrients, and yes, it can be. As I pointed out earlier, a vegan diet can be healthy or unhealthy depending upon its application. Any diet made up of processed food is going to be bad for you. If you are considering moving into being a full-time vegan, you might be concerned about how to get adequate calcium, protein, zinc, omega-3 and vitamin B_{12} in your diet. It can be difficult and involves an understanding of nutrition in order to get a full spectrum of the nutrients you need. A vegetarian diet, where you also eat dairy and eggs, is less likely to result in these deficiencies. If you intend to eat meat, fish and dairy for part of the week, however, you should be consuming sufficient quantities of those nutrients.

Surprisingly, it is not just a vegan diet that can lead to nutritional deficiencies. Data from 2015 showed that the average family in the UK eats four times more processed or packaged food than fresh food, which could explain why many people have low levels of selenium, magnesium and iron, iodine and vitamin D.

This chapter outlines the micronutrients the body needs and the foods they are found in so that you can choose your foods wisely.

Minerals

Calcium is the most abundant mineral in our body. It is needed for the formation and maintenance of bones and teeth. Many people believe we get our most of calcium from animal products, particularly eggs, butter, beef and dairy; however, the most usable (known as 'bioavailable') form is found in green leafy vegetables. These are also rich in magnesium, which helps with the absorption of calcium, as well as vitamin K, which helps with bone density. We also need vitamin D and phosphorus in order to absorb and utilise calcium correctly. Calcium is found in nuts, seeds and some plant milks, such as almond and coconut milks.

Chromium plays an important role in balancing blood sugars by working with insulin to help push glucose out of the blood and into the cells, so sufficient amounts are especially important for anyone with insulin resistance or type-2 diabetes. This is also an important micronutrient for anyone who wants to lose weight and manage their sugar cravings. The best sources of chromium are broccoli, shellfish, pears, Brazil nuts, tomatoes and grapes.

Copper is a mineral that helps to support a healthy metabolism. It is especially needed for energy and is involved in the transportation of iron. There has been some research that shows improvements in certain neurological conditions such as Parkinson's and Alzheimer's disease, when supplemented with copper. Copper can help to reduce inflammation, especially joint pain caused by arthritis. Liver is one of the best forms of copper, but you can also get it from a variety of plant sources such as shiitake mushrooms, quinoa, kale, almonds, chia seeds and cashew nuts.

Iodine plays a vital role in healthy thyroid function. Iodine is also useful for conditions such as fibromyalgia, muscle weakness and pains, all of which can be signs of an iodine deficiency. When you think of iodine-rich foods, seafood such as oily fish and sea vegetables such as seaweed (the richest being kelp) usually come to mind, but it can also be found in natural yogurt, milk and eggs. You can also get small amounts of iodine from fruit and vegetables, such as potatoes, prunes, strawberries and cranberries.

Iron is needed to transport oxygen around the body, and a deficiency can cause anaemia and fatigue. If you increase your iron intake, ensure you also increase your vitamin C intake, as this is needed to utilise the iron efficiently. Iron is found in red meats, particularly liver, while vegan sources include nuts, seeds, beans, whole grains and green leafy vegetables. The good news is it is also found in dark chocolate.

Magnesium is vital for health and is the second most abundant mineral in our body. Magnesium works in balance with calcium, helping to combat stress and easing muscle tension. In fact, magnesium is essential in the body for energy synthesis right through to the metabolism of carbohydrates and protection of our heart health. More magnesium deficiencies are being found today, especially in woman. This is due to our highly processed diet and over-farmed soil. The most magnesium-rich foods are kelp, wheat bran, almonds, brewer's yeast, buckwheat, Brazil nuts, cashews and molasses, but you will also find lower levels in green leafy vegetables, peanuts, millet, rye, tofu, walnuts, pecans, coconut, brown rice, figs, dried fruit, avocado and hard cheese. Note that boiling vegetables can cause magnesium (and other vitamins and minerals) to leach out, so I recommend steaming or stir-frying.

Manganese is involved in many chemical processes within the body, from balancing hormones and cholesterol to the formation of bones, fighting free radicals (as described on page 19) reducing inflammation and improving cognitive function. Manganese absorption can be disrupted in the body by a number of factors, including medications such as birth control pills or by consuming phytates and oxalates (see box below). High alcohol consumption can also reduce the body's ability to absorb manganese. Manganese is found in many foods, but the richest sources are from plants, such as nuts, seeds, pulses and green leafy vegetables.

Reducing anti-nutrients in food

Anti-nutrients are substances that can bind to some minerals and nutrients, impairing their absorption in the body. They include phytates, antioxidant compounds that are found in pulses (peas, beans and lentils), whole grains, seeds and coffee; and oxalates, an organic acid found in spinach, rhubarb, beetroot, peanuts and wheat bran. It is possible to decrease the amount of anti-nutrients, for example by using sprouted grains and adequately cooking pulses, but you can also combine foods to increase absorption and utilisation of certain nutrients. Eating plenty of foods rich in vitamin C such as strawberries and citrus foods, for example, can counteract the blocking effect of phytates.

Phosphorus is the third most abundant mineral in the body and, as we saw earlier, it plays a key role in the absorption of calcium to help build bones and teeth, as well as being required for metabolism and energy, utilisation and absorption of macronutrients, cellular growth and repair, nerve and muscle contractions, balancing hormones and the removal of waste from the kidneys. The best foods containing phosphorus include beef, fresh tuna, dairy products and eggs, as well as vegan sources: seeds, beans, green leafy vegetables and almonds.

Potassium is the fourth most abundant mineral in the body and works with sodium in helping to regulate fluids and minerals within the body. The majority of our potassium is found in our cells. It is involved in transporting nutrients and waste in and out of the cells. It also plays an important role in nerve and muscle communications, helping the nerve impulses that cause our muscles to contract. We get the most potassium from fruit and vegetables, with the best sources being beans, avocados, sun-dried tomatoes, sweet potatoes, green leafy vegetables, bananas and apricots.

Selenium plays a key role in boosting the immune system and has also been shown to help reduce inflammation, cardio-vascular disease and even cancer. It can also help to optimise thyroid function. Deficiencies in selenium are being found in many people today, and this is believed to be due to soils where the vegetables are grown being depleted of the mineral, as well as our processed Western diet. Natural sources of selenium include eggs, liver and oily fish, with vegan sources being Brazil nuts, sunflower seeds and chia seeds.

Zinc is an antioxidant that helps to support the immune system, aiding protein synthesis, maintaining sexual health, and playing a vital role in supporting a healthy heart. Processed foods and high-sugar diets can lead to a deficiency in zinc. Zinc is found in lean protein, especially lamb and beef, dairy, eggs and seafood, with vegan sources being nuts, seeds, cocoa, chickpeas and whole grains.

Vitamins

Vitamin A is a fat-soluble vitamin and antioxidant. It is important for our eyesight as well as supporting the immune system. It maintains healthy skin, balances hormones and protects against free-radical damage. Ensure that you have adequate levels of zinc and iron (see above), as deficiencies in these can deplete vitamin A. This vitamin comes in two forms: retinol and carotenoids. Retinol is found only in animal products, such as liver, eggs, cheese and yogurt. The body can produce its own vitamin A, however, when you eat orange or yellow foods, which contain carotenoids. These are, for example, carrots, mangoes, papayas and sweet potatoes.

Vitamin B$_1$ (thiamine) All B vitamins work very closely together and most play a role in energy production. Thiamine is vital for a healthy nervous system as well as for heart health. Thiamine also helps with the breakdown of protein. It is found in pork and liver, as well as vegan sources: nutritional yeast flakes, macadamia nuts, whole grains, lentils and beans. People who have a heavily processed diet could find themselves deficient in vitamin B1.

Vitamin B$_2$ (riboflavin) is another key player in energy, as well as in the production of white blood cells, and it protects against free radicals. It has also been shown to help with migraines.

Riboflavin works closely with thiamine (vitamin B_1) and niacin (vitamin B_3). Riboflavin can be affected by a low thyroid, adrenal stress and excessive alcohol consumption. You can boost your B_2 by eating dairy products, especially natural yogurts, oily fish and red meat, with green leafy vegetables, such as spinach and broccoli, being the best vegan sources.

Vitamin B_3 (niacin) is needed to maintain a healthy heart, brain and skin and to balance blood sugar. It also plays a key role in helping to keep cholesterol levels balanced and could help to reduce triglyceride levels. The highest concentrations of niacin come from meat and fish sources, such as liver, red meat and oily fish, although you can also find quite a high level in sunflower seeds.

Vitamin B_4 (choline) is vital for fat absorption and utilisation as well as for liver health. It also plays a role in brain health, helping with mental clarity, concentration and mood. You will find it in liver, salmon and egg yolks, while the vegan sources are cauliflower, chickpeas and split peas.

Vitamin B_5 (pantothenic acid) plays a key role in energy production and can also help to balance blood sugar and cholesterol levels, as well as supporting the nervous system. Pantothenic acid is mostly found in red meat, but you can also find it in eggs. Vegan sources include sunflower seeds, portobello mushrooms, avocado, broccoli and pulses.

Vitamin B_6 (pyridoxine) is needed for the breakdown of proteins and plays a vital role in energy production. It also works alongside iron, aiding the transportation of oxygen and maintaining heart health. B_6 also works well alongside magnesium and vitamin E in relieving premenstrual tension (PMT) and mild depression. Liver is a rich source, and vegan sources are whole grains, brown rice and pulses.

Vitamin B$_7$ (biotin) Like all B vitamins, B$_7$ plays a role in energy production and is also important for digestion and the metabolism of fats, carbohydrates and protein, for cardiovascular health and the nervous systems. Biotin also helps to maintain and repair hair and nails. The richest sources are liver, eggs and oily fish such as salmon, and cheese; the vegan sources are avocado and yeast.

Vitamin B$_9$ (folic acid) is known mostly for its importance in pregnancy, due to its role in the development of the foetus (it is essential for cellular formation and DNA replication). The best sources of folate are found in liver, but you can also find it in green leafy vegetables, such as spinach, broccoli and Brussels sprouts, and in avocado and lettuce. Food manufacturers now fortify foods with folic acid, so it is also found in processed cereals and breads. Our bodies absorb and utilise natural folate better than synthetic folic acid sources, however.

Vitamin B$_{12}$ (cobalamin) deficiency can cause anaemia, fatigue and depression, and has even been linked to dementia. The best sources are found in liver, red meat, chicken and oily fish. You can also find B$_{12}$ in dairy products. Vegans are especially prone to Vitamin B$_{12}$ deficiency, as the richest sources are found in animal products, although a very small amount is found in some vegetables, yeast spreads and fortified cereals. If you are vegan and concerned about B$_{12}$, I advise taking a good-quality supplement daily.

Vitamin C is needed to keep the immune system in tiptop condition as well as for collagen formation, wound healing, gum health and cardiovascular health. Vitamin C also has great antioxidant properties, helping to mop up free radicals and reduce toxins and inflammation. You need vitamin C to utilise iron, so if you are anaemic, ensure you have adequate amounts of both. Cooking can destroy vitamin C, so it is important to try to get some raw sources into your diet every day. Opt for handfuls of berries (especially strawberries), citrus fruits, cherries, green leafy vegetables, peppers and melon.

Vitamin D A deficiency can affect the immune system, respiratory system (especially creating incidences of asthma) and contribute to depression, heart disease, multiple sclerosis, diabetes and even cancer. Vitamin D helps to lower blood pressure and to keep us calm and less anxious. It has even been shown to help the body break down stubborn fat cells. There are more incidences of people with low vitamin D levels today than in the past, mainly because we no longer spend so much time outdoors in the sun. You can get some vitamin D from foods such as oily fish and eggs (and it is added to some cereals and spreads), but studies have shown that the conversion from sunlight is much more powerful and has more of an impact on health. I would advise spending 20 minutes per day in the sunshine during the summer and taking a vitamin D_3 supplement during the winter months, as we do not get enough sunshine in the UK to top up our vitamin D naturally.

Vitamin E is a fat-soluble vitamin and, as a powerful antioxidant, it helps to protect the body from free-radical damage. It also helps to ease PMT, heals the skin, reduces cholesterol, balances the hormones and protects against cardiovascular disease. Vitamin E works best alongside vitamin C and selenium (see page 26). The best sources of vitamin E are sunflower seeds, almonds and hazelnuts. You can also find it in fish oils, olive oil and almond oils, avocados, mangos and butternut squash.

Vitamin K is needed for blood clotting and wound healing, a healthy nervous system and bone health. The richest sources of vitamin K are green leafy vegetables, particularly Swiss chard, kale, broccoli and spinach. You can also find it in tomatoes, olive oil, parsley and pepper.

Fibre

A plant-based diet is packed with fibre. We often think of fibre as a way to keep our bowels working properly, bulking out the stools and helping with the transition through the body, but fibre does more than simply aid our bowel movements.

There are two kinds of fibre: soluble and insoluble. Soluble fibre attracts water, bulking out the food into a gel-like substance that can help lower cholesterol, stabilise blood sugars, decrease fat absorption and feed our healthy bacteria, allowing it to thrive. Soluble fibre also helps us feel fuller for longer. Insoluble fibre helps with the transition of stools through the body by absorbing water, bulking out our stools and preventing constipation. Complex carbohydrates, as explained in Chapter 1, contain both soluble and insoluble fibre, and both play a role in slowing down the rate of digestion because the body has to work harder to digest and extract the nutrients from the food. This makes us feel fuller for longer. Fibre can also help to lower cholesterol and keep the heart healthy. Beta glucan, a type of fibre found in oats, has been shown to help lower cholesterol and protect the body from LDL damage.

Having covered the basics of nutrition, let's look at how that information translates to what foods you should choose.

Chapter 3

Nourishing Choices

We are constantly reading about food-health scares, so it can be hard to know what to believe, or indeed what to buy, to eat healthily. I am often asked what the healthiest diet is, and my answer is always the same: a real-food diet. How you adapt this diet of real food is down to your health, needs and wants, as everyone is different.

As we have seen, this book focuses on eating natural food, packed with antioxidant-boosting vegetables, good fats and quality protein sources. It is all about flexibility and the promotion of a diet that suits each individual's needs, while ensuring optimal health benefits. You might want to use this book as a stepping stone towards a vegan diet, or maybe you are focusing more on the health aspects of adding more plant-based meals to your diet while mixing in some omega-3-rich fish oils, meat and dairy. Whether you are moving towards becoming vegan or you simply want to add more of those healthy plant-based meals to your diet, you should not deviate from opting for the best-quality food you can afford, in its most natural state. The following guidance will help you to pick and choose foods to suit your own diet while focusing on a real-food diet and increasing your consumption of plant-based food.

Fruit and vegetables

As I stated early in this book, we get a wide range of nutrients from fruit and vegetables – nature has certainly provided well for us. As I touched upon on page 20, fruit and vegetables also provide a wide range of antioxidants, all of which help to feed, strengthen and support the body, as well as helping us to fight infection and clear our body of toxins and free radicals.

Phytonutrients are the plant chemicals. They actively fight against, and protect us from, damaging toxins in our body that create free radicals, which can damage our cells and even change the DNA of the cell. These phytonutrients can be classed into groups, including flavonoids, carotenoids, curcuminoids, lignans and sulphides, to name just a few. Each of these groups play a vital role in our health. It is not important to understand the complexities of each group, but it demonstrates why we need to feed our body a variety of colourful fruit and vegetables in order to get a range of phytonutrients to protect us from cellular damage.

There are varying reports on the quantity of fruit and vegetables we should be consuming. Public Health England promotes five portions a day, based on evidence from the World Health Organization recommendation of eating at least 400g of fruit and vegetables per day to help lower the risk of serious health problems such as heart disease, cancer and strokes. However, a study by Imperial College London recommends ten portions a day (800g), as it was shown that this can reduce the chance of a stroke by up to a third and the risk of heart disease by 24 per cent. The study suggested that if everyone ate 800g a day, it could prevent 8 million premature deaths worldwide. The one thing we all agree on is the need to include more vegetables in our diet!

Although most people are aware of the need to consume at least five portions of vegetables and fruit a day, many are confused about portion size and what foods are included. When I was working with a school a few years ago, teaching healthy eating, I was horrified when the teacher told me that she thought five a day was a maximum! I have lost count of the number of clients who include potatoes in their five a day. Some were including chips, others orange squash, and even tomato ketchup. Food manufacturers are cashing in on this confusion. I have seen endless sugary snack products, especially aimed at children, labelled as part of your five a day. It appears, then, we are listening to the message but making our own assumptions on how to execute it.

Vegetables are often neglected in favour of fruit, because people enjoy the sweetness and convenience of a piece of fruit for a snack, but we need to put more focus on vegetables and less on fruit. Fructose, although a natural fruit sugar found in fruit, does come with some health warnings.

The fruit containing the least amount of fructose are strawberries, raspberries, blueberries, lemons, plums, peaches, coconut and cantaloupe melon. Banana, grapes, mango, pineapple, pear, apple and kiwi all contain the highest amounts – banana and grapes being the highest of all.

Look at fruit as nature's candy and eat it in its whole form, not as a juice or when dried. Eating a whole fruit means that you are also eating some fibre, which slows down the digestion of the fructose. In contrast, if you drink your fruit in a juice, there is no fibre to break down, and, as a result, a high concentration of fructose floods the liver. Fructose is converted directly to fat by the liver. The higher incidences of fatty liver disease today might be caused by the consumption of large amounts of fructose. We are consuming more fruit juices and smoothies believing these are healthier alternatives to processed drinks. While they are natural, they are pure sugar, and can contain more sugar than a glass of cola, so they should be more of an occasional treat rather than an everyday drink. Food manufacturers are also adding fructose to our foods in the form of fruit concentrates and high-fructose corn syrup.

Pulses

Also called legumes, pulses are a staple of the vegan diet, providing protein and fibre. They include lentils, split peas and beans, such as chickpeas, butter beans, red kidney beans and haricot beans. You might be surprised to know that the peanut is also a legume and not a nut.

Pulses have been shown to help balance cholesterol, regulate energy levels and aid the digestion. The fibre in pulses helps the transition of food through our digestive system and bulks up our stools (see Fibre on page 31). Pulses are also rich in nutrients such as magnesium, phosphorus, manganese, iron and potassium.

Remember, however, that pulses do not deliver a complete protein, so if you are a full-time vegan, you need to think about adding a variety of protein sources, such as quinoa (which is a seed and sometimes known as a pseudo-grain), to gain the essential amino acids to make a complete protein source.

Pulses contain phytic acid, which can negatively affect the absorption of calcium, iron and manganese if you consume too many or rely too much on a diet rich in pulses, grains and cereals. You can limit the phytic acid, however, by sprouting the pulses, and this not only limits the phytic acid but also increases the nutritional content.

You must also ensure that you cook your pulses thoroughly, especially red kidney beans, which contain phytohemagglutinin, which is toxic when consumed in high levels. This is removed in cooking by rapidly boiling the pre-soaked beans for 10 minutes before simmering them until tender. Tinned beans are already cooked to this level.

You will find more information on the individual pulses and their nutritional benefits in Chapter 5.

Nuts and seeds

In the past we were always told to be wary of nuts because of their high fat content, but nuts and seeds are little powerhouses of nutrients, and we should include them in our diet. They contain fibre, protein, magnesium, manganese and healthy fat. A handful of nuts a day, such as almonds, has been shown to help lower cholesterol and the risk of developing heart disease.

The nutritional content of nuts and seeds varies depending on the type, so it is advisable to eat a selection. I have detailed more about the nutritional values for each individual nut and seed in Chapter 5.

Grains

When choosing grains, opt for the healthiest grains possible. Organic is a must to limit your exposure to agro-chemicals and genetically modified grains. Go for the best quality and the most natural, unprocessed option. I recommend buckwheat, spelt, quinoa, oats, brown rice and wild rice. Grains can raise your blood sugar level, so limit them if you are overweight or you are insulin resistant (in other words you have problems with blood sugar levels, you are pre-diabetic or you are type-2 diabetic).

Certain grains possess healthy qualities, and oats is one of the main ones. It can help to mop up toxins, so eating oats is especially helpful if you have an upset stomach. As we saw earlier, the beta glucan fibre found in oats helps to lower cholesterol and protect the body from LDL damage. Oats also contain a bioactive compound called avenanthramide, which can help to prevent fat from forming in the arteries, thereby reducing the risk of heart attack and strokes.

Oats and brown rice both increase levels of the amino acid, tryptophan, in the blood. Tryptophan produces serotonin (sometimes known as the feel-good hormone), which helps to regulate our mood.

Other grains have health benefits:

- Brown rice, spelt, quinoa and buckwheat are all good sources of manganese, potassium, magnesium, fibre and B vitamins.
- Spelt is also a good source of iron and zinc.
- Quinoa is a great protein source, containing all 20 amino acids.

Wheat and gluten

I am seeing more health problems in my clinic, most of which are eased once wheat is removed from a client's diet. It never fails to surprise me how eliminating wheat from the diet can help so many things, ranging from skin conditions such as acne, eczema and psoriasis, to gut health such as IBS, inflammation and migraines, to name but a few. Gluten is a protein and is an anti-nutrient. It is one of the most difficult to digest plant proteins and is known to cause digestive problems, allergic reactions and autoimmune issues, as well as migraines, fatigue and joint pain in some individuals.

Why, then, have many of us become intolerant to wheat? I believe the processed wheat we consume now is very different from the wheat we ate years ago. The modern strains of wheat have high levels of gluten and are heavily processed and drenched in agrochemicals, all of which can contribute to intolerances. This is made worse by our fragile gut biomes (as outlined briefly on page 51) and compromised immune systems.

Wheat and gluten can impact our health in many ways, ranging from raising blood sugars, laying down fat, lowering the immune system, compromising our digestive tract and causing inflammation, and they can even speed up the ageing process. Gluten- and wheat-free products are not desirable as alternatives, however, because they are all very processed and packed with sugar, other carbohydrates and starch. I prefer to buy organic spelt or buckwheat as this has less impact on our health, but in following a vegan diet it is not necessary to go gluten-free unless you wish to.

Mixing it up

The recipes in this book are all vegan, encouraging you to explore adding more plant-based foods at least two or three times a week. As the emphasis is on health and real food, we also need to look at the other foods in our diet of the part-time vegan: meat, fish, eggs, dairy, sugar and oils.

Meat

You might not want to eat meat for environmental reasons, or you might feel it is better to avoid it due to the health scares you may have read about. One often quoted study, The China Study, published in 2005, advocates a diet free from animal products as the key to good health, but, just like all studies, there is plenty of room for argument on both sides. Having read the study, my own conclusion is that animal-derived food is not to blame for our declining health; instead I would lay the blame firmly on the highly processed diets so many people eat.

If we look at the world's healthiest and longest living communities, we will find they live on a more plant-based diet, but they also avoid processed foods. The traditional Mediterranean diet is predominantly plant-based, and filled with healthy oils, but it also includes oily fish, dairy and occasional meat – again, the key is real food.

Cancer scares

The World Health Organization has recommended that we avoid processed meats due to an increase risk in colon cancer; however, the fault is not with the meat, but the processing, as well as the added fillers, chemicals, additives and sugars in the meat. Meat is not unhealthy; it is what manufacturers do to the meat that makes it of poor quality. It also stands to reason that those who eat a lot of processed meats are also more likely to have a processed diet generally. Furthermore, we should consider the state of our colons, as poor gut health can lead to an increased risk of tumours.

A study by the University of Leeds in 2018 compared rates of distal bowel cancer (in the part of the bowel that stores faeces) in 32,000 women who took part in the study, which lasted for 17 years. The researchers focused on rates of cancer in vegetarian and in meat and/or dairy diets and found that there was no evidence to link meat to an increase in colon or rectum cancer, but they also found that a vegetarian diet offered a protection against distal bowel cancer.

Over-cooking our meat, especially when we blacken the meat over a barbecue or on a griddle, can release harmful compounds, called heterocyclic amines and polycyclic aromatic hydrocarbons. These are chemicals that are formed when muscle meat is cooked at very high temperatures, or when it is exposed to smoke (such as barbecuing). These compounds have been linked to cancer in animals, although there is firm evidence showing that exposure to cooked/barbecued meats definitively causes cancer in humans. It is something we all need to be mindful of, and to treat our food with respect to limit our exposure.

I recently read in the *Lancet* about a South American tribe, the Tsimane, who are considered to have the healthiest hearts in the world, and yet they had high inflammatory markers in their bodies (these markers show inflammation, which can be from something simple such as an infection or an increased risk of heart attack or serious degenerative diseases). The Tsimane people live in the Bolivian Amazon and are the ultimate hunter–gatherers. They eat game, fish, plantain, rice, nuts and fruit. The report talks about their diet being low in saturated fats, and it suggests that this is the reason why they are healthy; I would argue once again, however, that it has more to do with the fact they have a diet of real food, free from processing.

Saturated fat

When discussing meat we need also to mention saturated fat. The need to reduce saturated fat consumption is often cited as a reason why many people opt to go vegan; however, as we saw on page 13, meat doesn't contain only saturated fats. It also contains polyunsaturated and monounsaturated fats – the fats that are considered to be healthy.

Humans have eaten meat for thousands of years, yet it is only in the last 40–50 years that we have seen the dramatic increase in cancer, heart disease, diabetes and other degenerative diseases. We could blame meat, but more realistic culprits would be food manufacturing, agrochemicals and industrial farming. We also need to consider how the animal has been raised, what it has been fed and the quality of its food – after all, we are what we eat. I would always recommend organic, grass-fed meat, the best quality you can afford, to ensure your meat is in its purest form. Meat is packed with protein, magnesium, potassium, zinc, iron, vitamins E and B vitamins, including B_6 and B_{12}. You can get protein from vegan sources – for example pulses, vegetables, nuts and some grains such as oats, quinoa and buckwheat – but you would have to consume a larger quantity of the vegan source, as well as a mixture of foods, to gain the correct amounts of the individual amino acids needed for health (see page 7).

Fish

You have, no doubt, seen scare stories about the high levels of pollutants and toxins in our fish and farmed salmon; however, oily fish contains omega-3 fats which, as we have seen, are vital for good health, so I do believe that these health benefits outweigh the potential negatives.

The popularity of the Mediterranean-style diet demonstrates this. Italy, for example, is one of the healthiest countries in the world. I highly recommend you watch a film called *The Big Fat Fix*, which focuses on the small village of Pioppi in Southern Italy. In the film, leading cardiologist Dr Aseem Malhotra and Donal O'Neill explore what makes the village residents live a long and very healthy life. Their diet is natural, plant-based with oily fish and small amounts of dairy and meat but, crucially, they put much more emphasis on having a good lifestyle – experiencing more time outside in the sun, less stress with more relaxation and generally enjoying life. Ikaria in Greece also has some of the world's lowest rates of mortality; their diet is similar to that of Pioppi. You can also look at communities such as the Okinawans, whose traditional diet is primarily plant based with oily fish and healthy fresh soy. However, this is changing as these traditional diets are becoming more westernised, and this had a direct impact on life expectancy.

On page 14 I explained about the health properties of omega-3 fats found primarily in fish. The richest sources of omega-3 fish come from oily fish such as wild salmon, trout, mackerel, sardines, fresh tuna and herring. Omega-3 fat not only protects the heart and joints but it is also anti-inflammatory and has been shown to relieve a number of conditions, including depression, cognitive issues and cancer. Omega-3 also has an anti-clotting effect, helping to keep your blood flowing. Studies have shown that those with a higher blood level of omega-3 are a third less likely to die of heart disease. Oily fish also contains some vitamin D, vitamins A and B_2, phosphorus, selenium, calcium, protein, iron, zinc and iodine.

If you aim is to be fully vegan and wish to avoid eating fish, you can boost your omega-3 levels by eating nuts and seeds, and by adding flax oil to your diet. Flaxseeds and oil contain omega-3 in the form of alpha linolenic acid (ALA), however, so it is important to keep your consumption of omega-6 fats low, as explained on page 14.

Dairy products

I grew up on a dairy farm, where the milk would be brought into the kitchen in a jug straight from the cow, and although I have never really liked milk, I do eat some dairy, such as cheese, cream and yogurts, as well as plant-based 'dairy' products. Some people worry about hormones in our dairy products and meat products, and while these are not currently used in the UK, antibiotics and added chemicals are. However, these worries are alleviated once you opt for organic versions.

Dairy can cause some health issues; for example, respiratory and recurrent ear infections (in children) and eczema can often be eased by eliminating dairy while supporting the gut with good quality probiotics. Some menopausal women might find that they lose weight more easily if they stop eating dairy foods. It is worth noting, however, that you might only be intolerant to the lactose in the milk, so it is worth exploring the lactose-free milks, cheeses and yogurts that are now available.

Plant-based milks are popular with people who are making this switch, and who are looking for a healthier alternative. There are some fantastic dairy alternatives available, but some are quite heavily processed and contain sugar and fructose, and are therefore far from healthy. Always read the label carefully and avoid any sweetened with natural fruit, apple juice or similar.

If you eat dairy, opt for dairy in its more natural state: organic full-fat/whole milk, full-fat organic natural yogurt and natural cheeses such as brie, camembert, stilton and so on (as opposed to those made with emulsifiers, vegetable oils and whey). The fat is essential for good health, and, as stated earlier regarding meat, saturated fat is not a health concern. Removing the fat not only alters the quality of the food but also its nutritional values. Milk is packed with protein, calcium, iodine and vitamins B_2 and B_{12}.

Eggs

For many years we were fed the message that eggs raised our cholesterol. We now realise that natural sources of cholesterol from our food do not increase the risk of heart disease. Eggs, especially egg yolks, are little powerhouses of nutrients and as near as we can get to a complete food. They contain some omega-3 fatty acids, more so if they are free-range, as well as selenium, phosphorus, vitamin A, the B vitamins such as B_2, B_9 and B_{12}, and carotenoids such as lutein and zeaxanthin, which can help to protect us against macular degeneration and glaucoma. Eggs are also great for diabetics or those with insulin resistance and obesity, as they keep you full and suppress a ghrelin response (the hormone that makes you crave more food). They also contain choline, which can help to reduce a fatty liver and some neurological conditions such as dementia and depression. Just like meat, I would opt for organic, free-range eggs.

Vegans can make their own 'eggs' to use in baking or binding foods, such as nut roasts or burgers. You can use flaxseeds or chia seeds blended with water and left to thicken into a paste, or mashed banana or apple purée.

Sugar and refined carbohydrates

I cannot emphasise enough how important it is to limit the amount of sugar and refined carbohydrates we consume. I am passionate about this, having written three books on the subject. Today, there are epidemic levels of type-2 diabetes, obesity, heart disease, fatty liver disease, Alzheimer's disease and other inflammatory conditions, all of which can be attributed to a diet high in sugar and our addiction to refined carbohydrates.

It is quite hard for vegans, especially those reliant on processed foods, to keep their carbohydrates and sugar in check. One of the arguments for veganism is a lower BMI (body mass index), but it is possible to be vegan *and* overweight, especially if your diet is very carb heavy. Also, be aware of the new phenomenon called TOFI: thin outside, fat inside. This is due to a high intake of sugar and, in particular, fructose, flooding the body and causing it to lay down more fat in the liver and around the vital organs (known as visceral fat). Opting for real food helps dramatically. Remember to choose vegetables in preference to fruit to avoid too much fructose in your diet.

Some food manufacturers and food bloggers have recognised the need to reduce sugar, but are focusing on refined sugar. Sadly, our body doesn't differentiate between refined or unrefined sugars: it breaks them down in exactly the same way. Honey, molasses, maple syrup, dates, coconut sugar and agave syrup are all sugars, and they spike blood sugar levels, and therefore an insulin response, as well as delivering high levels of fructose. Eating these foods is just a sideways step. They still cause a ghrelin response, and fructose also turns off the leptin response – the hormone that tells our brain when we are full. That 'natural' date-based snack bar that you might choose as a healthy alternative will perpetuate your cravings, raise your blood sugars and flood your liver with fructose, so it is not quite as healthy as we might have been led to believe.

High-fructose sweeteners

Fructose has been shown to increase the production in the body of something called endogenous AGEs (advanced glycation end products), which has been linked to age-related and degenerative disorders. Those with high blood sugars also appear to produce more AGEs.

As explained earlier, fructose is processed by the liver and becomes converted to fats, which are stored in the liver, contributing to non-alcoholic fatty liver disease, as well as being pushed into the adipose tissue, contributing to obesity and its related conditions.

Fructose is also connected to oxidised LDL and to age-related and degenerative disorders. It can increase inflammation in the whole body and the risk of oxidative damage to the cells. It also increases uric acid production, which can lead to high blood pressure, gout and kidney stones.

Fructose stimulates the hunger hormone ghrelin, which growls at us to eat more, and it can also shut off our leptin response. It also has a detrimental effect on our looks, as it interferes with collagen production, causing the skin to lose elasticity and increasing the risk of wrinkles.

Your bowel health can be affected, too. Bad bacteria feed off of the sugars in your diet, particularly fructose. Poor bowel health not only affects your digestion and bowel habits but also lowers your immune system and can increase your risk of tumours. Poor bowel health also affects how your body deals with cholesterol.

My advice is to avoid anything high in fructose. This includes:

- **Agave Syrup**, which contains the most fructose of any of the 'natural' sugar replacements, with up to 97 per cent fructose. This is actually higher than high-fructose corn syrup!
- **Coconut sugar**, which is made up of sucrose, glucose and fructose. Because sucrose is 50 per cent glucose and fructose, if we add everything together, coconut sugar contains between 40 and 50 per cent fructose. This is very similar to standard sugar.
- **Dates** are used a lot to help sweeten desserts and baked goods. Date-based bars are advocated as healthy because they contain no refined sugar, or no *added* sugar, but don't be fooled, because these are packed with sugar and will raise blood sugars and flood your liver with fructose in exactly the same way.
- **Maple syrup** Many celebrity chefs are using maple syrup instead of sugar. Yes, maple syrup is natural, but your body still breaks it down in the same way as sugar, honey or brown sugar. Maple syrup is almost 100 per cent sucrose, which, just like table sugar, is made up of 50 per cent glucose and 50 per cent fructose. It will spike your blood sugar in exactly the same way as refined sugar.

Natural sweeteners

I prefer to avoid sugar and related high-fructose products, so I would advocate using erythritol, stevia or xylitol. These may sound scary and artificial, but they are from natural sources.

Erythritol blend This sugar alcohol is found in grapes and pears. Erythritol contains zero calories and does not affect blood sugar or insulin levels during or after consumption, making it safe for diabetics and for those following a low-carb diet. Unlike other sugar alcohols, such as xylitol, erythritol is well absorbed from the digestive tract, it passes into the urine and eliminated from the body, so it does not have a laxative side effect.

Stevia is a subtropical wild plant. The leaves of stevia contain glycosides whose sweetening power is between 250 and 400 times their equivalent in sugar. Stevia contains no calories and no carbohydrates. It does not raise blood sugar or stimulate an insulin response, so, for many, it is the preferred choice, as it is completely natural. Stevia is very sweet and the cheapest natural sweetener out of all three, but it does have a strange aftertaste, which is hard to control. I have found that liquid stevia has less aftertaste, but finding out whether you like it is really trial and error and depends on the brand you use. I use Sweetleaf Stevia drops – they are very good and have the least aftertaste. Always check the label to ensure it is pure stevia and not a blend of stevia with sugar.

Xylitol is a natural sugar alternative first discovered in birch wood. It has now been found in a host of other plants and fruits, such as sweetcorn and plums. Xylitol looks and tastes just like normal granulated sugar. It can, however, have a laxative effect in some people if eaten to excess. The laxative effect is caused because xylitol attracts water to it. This effect is different from one person to the next and can change as your body gets used to it. (You also need to keep xylitol, or any food made with it, well clear of dogs. As with grapes and chocolates, dogs metabolise xylitol quite differently to humans and it can be very dangerous for them, even in small amounts.)

Artificial sweeteners

I avoid artificial sweeteners, as I have read too many studies linking their use to mental-health problems and health complaints. There is now mounting evidence to show that artificial sweeteners are highly addictive and can increase your sugar cravings. They can also contribute to insulin resistance and diabetes and have been linked to headaches, hypertension, anxiety and even seizures.

Seed oils and margarines

Our consumption of man-made oils and margarines, and the variety of foods containing them, exposes us to an abundance of omega-6 and -9 oils and, as we have seen above, these are very inflammatory. Our fear of saturated fat has prompted us to consume more man-made and processed fats in the form of corn oil, safflower oil, sunflower oil, canola oil, rapeseed oil and palm oil, which are added to our everyday foods. As mentioned previously, the more omega-6 and omega-9 fats we consume, the harder it is for us to convert the omega-3 fat found in plant sources into the more active form of omega-3 (which is found in animal sources).

Not only are these man-made oils inflammatory but they are also usually highly processed, and some use genetically modified ingredients, altering the natural oils into a poor quality, toxic and often carcinogenic oil. These oils are not stable and are susceptible to changes once exposed to light, heat and oxygen.

In preference to seed oils I recommend that you choose instead good-quality pure olive oils (rather than olive oil mixed with other oils) in dark containers, coconut oil, flax oil and avocado oil. For cooking at high temperatures, I recommend using coconut oil, as it has a higher smoke point than olive oil and avocado oil, meaning that it is not damaged by heat. Use a good-quality extra virgin olive oil or flax oil for salad dressings.

If you want to be a part-time vegan, and are therefore not averse to using butter, you can use this. Butter is a pure, natural fat and far more stable than seed oils when heated, although not to high temperatures. You could also consider ghee, goose fat or even lard for frying, as these fats do not sustain damage, even at high temperatures.

Don't overlook your gut health

Poor diet, stress, smoking and erratic eating patterns not only affect the production of digestive enzymes and stomach acid but also play havoc with our natural bowel flora. Our digestive tract contains roughly 1.3kg of bacteria, both good and bad. We need the healthy (good) bacteria to thrive, as this helps to keep our immune system working well. Having a gut populated by bad bacteria, however, not only increases our risk of tumours (especially colorectal) but it also impacts on how well we absorb and utilise the nutrients we eat.

Good, healthy bowel flora plays a vital role in the removal of cholesterol. It also helps to balance blood sugars, helps us absorb and utilise antioxidants, supports our skin health (especially to improve acne), helps to control IBS, prevents candida and, due to its immune-boosting role, it can even help to prevent allergies. New research is also emerging to show how a healthy gut can help with obesity, depression and auto-immune diseases.

Some medications can alter our gut flora, including antibiotics, painkillers, and even the contraceptive pill.

Choose foods for a healthy gut microbiome

To enhance the good bacteria, we need to include foods that will create the right environment for our healthy bowel flora to thrive. These are the foods that contain prebiotics, such as those found in onions, garlic, leeks, artichokes, chicory root and seaweed, which help to improve our digestion, boost the immune system, reduce inflammation, balance hormones and help protect the heart. Garlic, in particular, has amazing health-promoting properties, especially in relation to bowel health. It is a natural antibiotic and anti-parasitic, and it also helps to prevent the formation of unhealthy gut bacteria. We also need to eat natural *probiotics* such as kefir, sauerkraut, kimchi, kombucha and natural yogurts, to help add to the essential friendly bacteria in our gut. You can also buy high quality probiotic capsules, which are especially good if your natural flora has been upset by overseas travel or medications such as antibiotics.

An alkaline diet is also great for our overall health. This is a diet that is low in acid-producing foods such as refined sugar, wheat, processed meats and some fresh meats, such as beef and pork, fizzy drinks and caffeine. A hydrating and alkalising diet will help to populate the bowel with friendly bacteria. An alkaline diet is also anti-inflammatory, which in turn helps to lower our risk of disease.

In addition to the prebiotic and probiotic foods mentioned above, there are a number of herbs and spices that have a positive effect on our bowel health:

- Cardamom is great to use if you suffer with IBS (inflammatory bowel syndrome) as it also contains anti-spasmodic properties.
- Cinnamon and cardamom have been shown to help prevent and reduce tumour growth.

- Cinnamon is anti-inflammatory as well as containing anti-microbial properties.
- Cloves can also help combat fungal infections, including *Candida albicans*.
- Cumin works well with turmeric to promote healthy gut flora.
- Fennel seeds aid digestion, and are particularly good for indigestion and constipation; they also have antispasmodic properties.
- Ginger is anti-inflammatory, anti-microbial and a great to help relieve nausea and poor digestion.
- Parsley is rich in vitamin C and carotenoids to help protect the intestinal wall.
- Peppermint can relieve bloating and indigestion as well as soothing and clearing the colon. It is also anti-viral, anti-bacterial and can reduce the risk of tumours.
- Turmeric, known to be a powerful anti-inflammatory due to the active compound called curcumin, is an excellent prebiotic.

In the next part I discuss about how to make economical choices when shopping, and how to build a store-cupboard suitable for a varied diet containing more plant-based foods.

Part II

THE SHOPPING ESSENTIALS

The chapters in this section contain the essentials for anyone starting off on a plant-based diet. I have tried to include all the foods I use on a daily basis, with descriptions of how and when to use it.

Chapter 4

A Healthy Diet Needn't Cost the Earth

We often hear the argument that only the rich can afford to eat a healthy diet, but really it can be economical to eat a good diet if done correctly. The way of eating that I promote is all about eating good food prepared from scratch and avoiding all the processed and junk foods. There are many ways to save money – they might seem like common sense, but they really are worth following, as they can save you time as well as money.

Quick-and-easy money-saving tips

Meal plans One of the best ways to save money is to plan ahead, and I don't just mean for one day. Knowing what you are going to eat for the week ahead is a great time and money saver. We are creatures of habit, repeating our food choices week by week. You will find that you need to prepare only two or three weekly meal plans and then rotate them. It is also worth planning your lunches, especially if you need working lunches to avoid the grab-and-go supermarket lunch meal deals.

Buy in bulk whenever you can You can always use your freezer to store any of the food bargains. Remember to label foods with the date.

Extend the life of your food by storing it correctly. You can buy preserving bags for fruit, potatoes and vegetables, which really does help to keep those foods fresh for longer. You can also vacuum pack your food. I use my freezer to store leftover foods and preserve anything I haven't had time to eat. Kitchen paper is a good absorber of moisture, which helps to preserve foods, so use it to line your vegetable and salad trays. I remove all my fruit and vegetables from their packaging before storing them in the fridge or in preserving bags.

Fruit and vegetables omit ethylene gas, which makes them spoil easily. If you pop a browning banana near other fruit, it will turn the fruit pretty quickly, so store fruit carefully. You can also buy gadgets to eliminate the gases.

Mushrooms are best stored in paper bags. If you're eating cheese on non-vegan days, this is best stored in waxed paper. Tomatoes and strawberries are better served at room temperature as it increases their flavour, but I store them in the fridge until needed. I store my nuts, seeds, pulses and flours, and so on, in glass jars.

Buy in season and explore your local markets for bargains. Buying in season means that there is often an abundance of a specific fruit or vegetable at any particular time, especially if you are lucky enough to be growing it yourself. I have joined local Facebook groups where we swap our own home-grown produce. It works well and can save a huge amount of money. But for people buying in the greengrocer, markets or supermarkets, you will still find produce is cheaper when in season.

Shop around I have found supermarkets such as Lidl and Aldi are much cheaper for pantry items such a nuts, fruit and vegetables than other supermarkets. Some supermarkets are now selling imperfect vegetables; although these are not organic, they might suit your budget more.

Join a cooperative There are loads around, such as Essential Trading Co-operative and Suma, where you can buy health food and store-cupboard foods in bulk or join forces with friends to share larger orders.

Look at organic delivery boxes They can save you money if you shop around. Some companies do introductory offers, and you can make some savings trying them out.

Shop online You are least likely to give in to impulse buys this way. It also saves quite a bit of time. We are all creatures of habit and tend to buy the same foods week in and week out. Most supermarkets store your favourite foods in one list, so often it is just a matter of quickly popping the items into your online trolley.

Buy a slow cooker I am a huge fan of the slow cooker. You simply chop the ingredients, throw them into the crock, add some stock, and away you go. When you return home in the evening, you have a meal ready with very little effort. You might be surprised at the variety of dishes you can make in your slow cooker – it doesn't always have to be soup and casseroles! I make cakes, jams, puddings, curries and chillies. I use a multicooker, which allows me to use the appliance in a variety of ways: to sauté, bake, roast, slow cook and steam. Most slow cookers also have a 'warm' facility, which is automatically switched on when it finishes cooking. This is invaluable, especially if you get home late, because it stops your dinner from being spoilt

Should you buy organic?

In an ideal world we would all be eating only organic food, but reality can be very different. It can be hard to get everything organic and, in some cases, it can double or even triple our food costs. Although there are people who believe that there is no benefit nutritionally from organic food, I think you can taste the difference. I also prefer the welfare standards that are required of organic meat, dairy and eggs.

Over 300 different pesticides are found on our foods, and most of these cannot be removed by washing them. When you look at the possible effects of pesticides and other agrochemicals on our food, it becomes quite scary. There are no current tests on the cocktail effect of all the chemicals we are exposed to on a day-to-day basis, from agrochemicals, household cleaners and air fresheners, right through to air pollution, chemicals used on our carpets and walls, and more. The Soil Association found pesticide residues in 43 per cent of British food items, such as fruit, vegetables, bread, dairy and meat, with many samples containing multiple pesticides. The more we learn about the damage agrochemicals can cause to our health, the less we tend to worry about the cost of buying organic. Personally, I think it is worth trying to get as much organic food as you can, but you could prioritise your organic purchases.

Fruit and vegetables

The same study in the *British Journal of Nutrition* also found that organic crops had 60 per cent more of the key antioxidants and lower levels of the toxic metal cadmium, than conventionally produced crops. According to the Pesticide Action Network UK (PAN UK), mushrooms, avocados and sweet potato have the lowest levels of pesticides, so these are fine to buy non-organic. Their list of foods to buy organic includes the following:

Apples
Apricots
Bananas
Berries, including raspberries and strawberries
Cherries
Citrus fruits such as oranges, lemons and limes
Cucumber
Grapes
Herbs
Pineapple
Pre-packed salad leaves
Spring greens and kale

For starchy foods and grains, high pesticide levels were found in oats, wheat, cereal bars, rice, bread, flour and crackers.

Chicken and eggs

If, as a part-time vegan, you are including chicken and eggs in your diet, I would urge you to buy organic. Many people opt for free-range believing it to be almost as good as organic, but the label organic means a bird should not contain any pesticides, hormones or antibiotics (or at least they should only be given to treat disease and not routinely given to prevent it), while free-range simply means that a bird can spend no more than 12 weeks inside, with a minimum space of 1 square metre for every nine hens. To be given organic status in the UK by the Soil Association, birds need to be raised to much higher welfare standards.

Dairy and meat

According to a 2014 study led by Professor Carlo Leifert, published in the *British Journal of Nutrition*, organic milk and meat contain 50 per cent more omega fatty acids than non-organic and there is a slightly lower concentration of saturated fats in organic meat. Organic milk contains 40 per cent more linoleic acid and has more iron, vitamin E and carotenoids. If you are eating dairy and meat on your non-vegan days, I recommend that you buy organic. These foods should be free from the routine use of antibiotics, have a higher standard of animal welfare and will be naturally grass-fed, free from pesticides and herbicides.

Soya

Soya is a very controversial food. In its natural state, it can have good health benefits when eaten in moderation, including being packed with hormone-balancing isoflavones; however, humans have stepped in and created a genetically modified monster. For this reason, I would only ever use organic soya products.

Waste not, want not

We are spending our hard-earned cash on buying the best food we can, yet in the UK we still waste a huge amount of food, with the average household throwing away about £700 a year in food waste. According to statistics, in 2015 the UK sent 7.3 million tonnes of food waste to landfill, all of which could have been eaten if we had shopped a little more wisely, planned ahead and stored the food correctly. I recently read an article discussing food waste; the UN's Food and Agriculture Organization stated that one-third of the food produced for human consumption is lost or wasted every year, amounting to 1.3 billion tonnes. This is made all the more shocking when we consider that there are nearly 8 million people in the world suffering from malnourishment.

Here are some tips to make the most of those odds and ends we all usually discard around the kitchen.

Bananas	No one likes a browning banana, but if you find they are starting to ripen too quickly, peel them and put chopped banana in a bag in the freezer. These can be used in smoothies, banana cake or puddings.
Coconut milk	Sometimes I have too much coconut milk to add to one dish. I freeze any leftovers in large ice-cube trays and just pop out a couple of cubes as and when I need them.
Nuts and seeds	Nuts and seeds can be frozen, but I tend to only buy what I need and store them in airtight jars.
Pulses	You can store pulses in their dried form for months. I have lots of Kilner jars in my kitchen and pantry filled with a variety of pulses. You can, of course, buy tinned pulses, but this does cost more. Instead, why not bulk cook, drain and then freeze, ready to add to your favourite recipe?

Ripe avocados	Scoop out the flesh of ripe avocados and mix with a touch of lemon or lime juice, then freeze. Once defrosted, use to make dips, chocolate mousse or a smoothie base.
Ripe tomatoes	Chop ripe tomatoes and freeze ready to use in tomato or pasta sauces. I prefer to slow-bake them in the oven with garlic and herbs and store them in jars with some olive oil.
Salads	Ensure you store salads correctly. I place salad leaves in a box and add a sheet or two of kitchen paper, as it absorbs any unwanted moisture. Raw tomatoes taste much nicer in a salad when they are at room temperature, but they do last longer if stored in the fridge.
Vegetables	You can freeze most vegetables. Alternatively, if you have any leftover vegetables, why not make a delicious soup or casserole, and then store it in the freezer as a nutritious homemade ready meal? Look at extending the life of your fruit and vegetables by using food-preserving bags. Lakeland sell some great ones for vegetables, such as a potato preserving bag, which is good not just for potatoes but also for any root vegetable. They also do banana bags, onion bags and vegetable bags. It is well worth considering extending the life of your produce.
Wine	If you have any wine left in the bottom of a bottle, you can it freeze into small portions ready to add to casseroles or pasta sauces.

Chapter 5

The Vegan Store-Cupboard

There are a few basic things that you will need to have in your store-cupboard when you begin cooking vegan meals. You may not be familiar with some of them, but most are available from leading supermarkets and health-food shops. I try not to use any obscure or unusual ingredients in my cooking. Anything I do recommend is used regularly throughout the book. I suggest that when you start out on plant-based eating you begin by looking at the recipes in the book that appeal to you and then make a list of the ingredients you will need, using this guide to help you. As you become more familiar with plant-based eating, you might want to build up your selection of foods as listed here.

The pantry essentials

These store-cupboard foods are my essentials and are available from good supermarkets and health-food stores.

Coconut Products

Coconut aminos Use this to add a great flavour to savoury dishes. Coconut aminos is a blend of coconut tree sap with organic sea salt. It is vegan, free from GMO and gluten-free. It can be used in a similar way to soy sauce, but without the associated health concerns of processed soy sauce. For a more economical choice opt for organic tamari, which is usually gluten-free too, or shoyu sauce.

Coconut cream I use this in cooking, such as in curries, as well as for desserts. When you want the cream from the top of a tin of coconut milk, pop the tin, upright, into the freezer for 1 hour to chill. This makes the cream more solid so that you can scoop it off.

Coconut flakes are like coconut shavings. They work well in my homemade granolas (page 93–4) and trail mix (page 226).

Desiccated coconut If you like to bake, you will find that this is useful because it is very fine and gives a nice coconut flavour. You can buy desiccated coconut in sweetened or unsweetened forms. I recommend you buy the latter.

Grains and flours

Almond flour (or ground almonds) Almond flour is much finer than ground almonds for using in cakes and it does give superior results, but, to be honest, I use ground almonds all the time, as they are far cheaper, and things still work out well. Ground almonds are also good added to soups, curries and nut roasts.

Buckwheat or spelt flour Buckwheat is actually a seed, not a grain, and is packed with antioxidants. It's an excellent alternative to wheat and is rich in rutin, a heart-healthy flavonoid. Spelt is a grain with similar credentials to wheat, but without the associated intolerance and gluten allergy issues. Spelt is also higher in copper, zinc, phosphorus and magnesium as well as vitamin B$_3$.

Coconut flour is more often used in low carb-diets and is a great alternative to carb-rich flours, if you wish to take the plant-based way of eating further than in this book and make cakes. It is also useful for those who are following a grain-free way of eating. It is a lot drier than other flours, however, absorbing up to ten times its weight, so you will need to make some adjustments to your baking if you use this.

Quinoa You might be concerned about finding sufficient protein sources when following a more plant-rich diet, but fear not, quinoa is a complete protein source. We think of quinoa as a grain, but it is actually a seed. It is also gluten-free. Use this as a direct replacement for rice, pasta or couscous to make your meal more nutrient dense. You will find simple instructions for how to cook quinoa on page 149.

Herbs and spices

There are no restrictions on herbs, spices and seasonings in a vegan diet, but I recommend that you check that any seasoning blends you buy don't have any added sugar. I use a lot of seasonings and make my own blends (see my harissa paste on page 241). My absolute staples are paprika, onion granules and garlic granules (not garlic salt), turmeric, oregano, thyme, basil, curry powder, chilli powder, chilli flakes and cinnamon. You can use fresh herbs; they are all wonderful but they are not always practical. (See also box page 84 for tips on freezing herbs.)

Natural sweeteners

As you may have noted previously in the book, I am passionate about a sugar-free way of eating. There is a lot of misinformation regarding sugar-free, however, and what might be the correct sweeteners to use in baking. Some people opt to be free of refined sugar, instead opting for maple syrup, agave or honey, but, as I explained on page 47, they are still sugars. I recommend using stevia, xylitol or erythritol, which are all from natural sources (you can read in more detail about natural sweeteners on pages 47–48).

Erythritol blend contains zero calories and does not affect blood sugar or insulin levels. Unlike xylitol (below), erythritol does not have a laxative side effect. I use Sukrin products, but you can also use Natvia brand. You can also buy icing sugar in these ranges.

Sukrin Gold is an Erythritol blend and a great alternative to brown sugar. I use it quite a lot to create a deeper sweet flavour. You can also buy this as a fibre syrup.

Stevia contains no calories and no carbohydrates. It is very sweet and the cheapest sweetener of the three described here. It does have a strange aftertaste, however. I use Sweetleaf Stevia drops: they are very good and have the least aftertaste. Always check the label to ensure it is pure stevia and not a blend of stevia with sugar.

Xylitol has 40 per cent less calories than sugar and less than 50 per cent of the available carbohydrates. The UK's leading brand of xylitol is Total Sweet, which is made from sustainable European birch and beech wood. It is available from most supermarkets.

Nut and seed butters

When buying a nut butter, always check the ingredients: it should contain only nuts, nothing else! I would also encourage you to make your own nut butters (page 238) and experiment by adding other healthy ingredients such as chia seeds or coconut.

Almond butter is useful for baking and savoury dishes. It is great when added to a hot curry.

Peanut butter can be very versatile for cakes, sweet dishes and savoury snacks, although I prefer other nut butters because they have higher nutritional values. As noted above, be very strict about the type of peanut butter you purchase.

Tahini is made from sesame seeds and is an essential ingredient of hummus (page 141), making a complete protein in combination with the chickpeas. Tahini is packed with B vitamins, magnesium, calcium and protein. It is also lovely on its own, or used as replacement for butter, or it can be good as a binder.

Nutritional yeast flakes

You may not have not heard of these. They look like the flakes you feed to fish, but they are packed with B vitamins. They give food a cheese flavour and you will find that they are used frequently throughout the book. I also use nutritional yeast flakes to create my own vegan Parmesan, which you can find on page 237. I buy them in a pot from health-food shops.

Nuts

I use a lot of nuts in my cooking, mostly almonds, pecan nuts, walnuts, hazelnuts, macadamia nuts and Brazil nuts. I also use fresh nuts and blend them to make nut butters and flours. Although I would normally urge you to buy in bulk, with nuts you have to be careful because they can go rancid and mouldy. If you want to buy them in bulk, you can store them in the freezer to help maintain their freshness, but I buy nuts in smaller quantities and store them in airtight glass jars.

Nuts are great to use in your own granola and nut bars (see pages 93–4 and 230). You can also make spicy nuts as a healthy replacement to crisps (see page 224).

You can 'activate' nuts to make their nutrients more easily absorbed by your body when eaten. This involves soaking them in water overnight, or in the case of some nuts, such as cashew nuts, a soak of about one to two hours. It is not necessary to do this in all cases, however, and I will let you know in individual recipes where this might be required.

Almonds I use a lot of almonds in my cooking (often ground almonds). They are higher in protein than walnuts and also contain higher levels of vitamin E and riboflavin, as well as manganese, magnesium and phosphorus.

Brazil nuts are one of the richest sources of selenium there is. They also contain good sources of magnesium, copper, phosphorus and manganese. Although they are great if you have a deficiency or want to support your thyroid health, it is possible to have too much selenium.

Cashew nuts are the most carb-rich of all the nuts, but they do contain good levels of protein, copper, zinc and magnesium.

Cashew nuts are useful for vegan cooking because they can be soaked to form a very creamy base, ideal for desserts and soups.

Hazelnuts are very high in manganese and provide a good source of copper, vitamin E, magnesium and B vitamins. They add richness to the flavour of homemade granola (page 93–4) and trail mix (page 226) and they can also be ground to make flour for a pastry base.

Macadamia nuts contain the most monounsaturated fatty acids of all the nuts. They are high in manganese, vitamins A and B, and iron. They are delicious roasted for 8 minutes and then coated in melted dark chocolate.

Peanuts Despite the name, peanuts are actually a legume and not a nut. Peanuts are popular snacks, but be careful that you are consuming only the best quality you can, without any added ingredients, oils or coatings. Peanuts deliver good quantities of copper, manganese and B vitamins. They also contain high levels of protein.

Pecan nuts are much sweeter than walnuts, with an almost toffee-like flavour. Like other nuts, pecan nuts are packed with manganese, copper, magnesium, zinc and B vitamins. They taste great sprinkled on top of coconut yogurt.

Pine nuts are a seed with a lovely nutty flavour. I sauté them in a little coconut oil to add to my salads, and they are also an essential ingredient in my homemade pesto (page 175).

Walnuts combined with mushrooms make an excellent vegan alternative to mince, and you will find several variations on the theme in this book (see page 180 for example). Walnuts contain vitamin E as well as omega-3 fats. They also supply good levels of manganese, copper, magnesium and phosphorus.

Oils

Coconut oil is a saturated fat, but it is a very healthy choice. It contains medium-chain fatty acids (MCFAs), making it easier to digest and process, as explained on page 15. Many people worry about overpowering food with a coconut taste, but it honestly doesn't do this. It can be tempting to buy cheap forms of coconut oil, such as copra, but it is heavily processed, is completely different to the organic, cold-pressed oil, and doesn't have the same health benefits.

Flax oil is packed with omega-3 fatty acids in the form of alpha linolenic acid (ALA), which is essential for vegans because they don't eat fish or take fish oils (as explained on page 14). Never heat flax oil, which would destroy the oil's amazing properties. Always buy your organic flax oil in a dark bottle and store it away from sunlight. Light, heat and oxygen will destroy its healthy properties. I use flax oil as a salad dressing and to make hummus (page 141).

Olive oil We all know about the benefits of olive oil and the Mediterranean-style diet. Olive oil is packed with anti-inflammatory compounds. It is mostly made of mono-unsaturated fatty acids, the most important being oleic acid, which has been shown to protect the heart and fight free-radical damage. It also contains about 14 per cent saturated and 11 per cent polyunsaturated fats. Buy the best quality you can afford, because some cheaper olive oils can often be a mixture of other oils. Unfortunately, even olive oil can change composition when heated at high temperatures, so I would prefer to use organic coconut oil when heating above a medium heat.

Pulses (peas, beans and lentils)

Most pulses are good sources of fibre and protein. They are a good staple for the vegan and vegetarian diet. Dried beans are the cheapest to buy in bulk, but remember that you will need to soak them overnight before cooking. A pressure cooker is very useful for cooking beans quickly because some, for example chickpeas, take a long time to cook until tender. They can be cooked in bulk and frozen. Lentils and split peas do not require soaking, however. You can also buy tinned pulses.

Butter beans are rich with potassium, fibre, iron and B vitamins. I don't use butter beans as often as chickpeas or cannellini beans, so I tend to buy these in tinned form.

Cannellini beans are rich in potassium and great to add to any casserole, soup or main meal. They have been shown to aid weight loss due to their ability to inhibit your body from absorbing carbohydrates quickly.

Chickpeas have a nutty taste and are great to add to dishes or to use as a base for burgers (page 205), falafels (page 108) and hummus (page 141). They absorb flavours well. Chickpeas are a good source of protein, fibre, manganese, copper, phosphorus, folate, iron and zinc. You can also retain the chickpea water (called aquafaba) from tinned chickpeas and use it to make desserts: whisk the chickpea water as you would egg whites, and add sweetener and vanilla extract to create your own vegan version of a delicious Pavlova.

Lentils I use red lentils, Puy lentils and brown lentils. Red lentils dissolve almost to nothing when cooked, and are good for thickeners and bulking, and for quick soups, and they are essential for dahls. I use Puy lentils more in salads, because they hold their shape well and their flavour really stands out. Brown lentils are good to add to casseroles, as they also hold their shape and they have a good flavour. Lentils are packed with fibre, protein, folate and manganese. They are also a good source of magnesium, B vitamins, zinc and copper. Lentils can be cooked from dried, without any soaking. I occasionally use tinned green lentils, which are quick and easy if you want to add instant protein to your meal.

Red kidney beans You can use these beans in many savoury dishes, but they are the best known for adding to a chilli. Kidney beans contain a good amount of magnesium, potassium, folate, iron, manganese, copper and phosphorus.

Split peas make great soups. I also like to use yellow split peas to make the traditional dish, pease pudding. They don't need to be soaked and can be added in dried form to any dish and cooked, just like lentils, although they do take longer than lentils.

Rice and pasta

Brown basmati rice is nutritionally superior to white rice. Both brown and white basmati rice contain almost identical levels of carbohydrates (brown rice is very slightly lower) but due to the additional fibre in brown basmati, you absorb these carbohydrates at a slower rate. Rice, whether white or brown, is not particularly high in protein, although it does contain a little, so it is important to combine it with another good protein source. I like to mix rice with quinoa. Brown rice also contains iron and a range of B vitamins.

Vegetable rice I am a huge fan of vegetable rice, made from finely chopped cauliflower (my favourite), broccoli or even beetroot.

I eat this now in preference to rice as I find that rice makes me feel a little bloated. I have added some recipes for you in the Side Dishes chapter and urge you to give it a go.

Wild rice, made from grasses, has a nutty flavour, and it also has slightly better credentials than brown basmati rice: it is rich in magnesium, manganese, phosphorus and B vitamins. It also contains antioxidants, such as phenolic acid – a naturally occurring phytonutrient that can help protect your heart.

Buckwheat and spelt pasta I prefer to limit the amount of pasta I consume so that my meals are not bulked out with carbohydrate, but if you do opt for pasta, ensure it is the most nutrient-rich source, such as buckwheat or spelt.

Pasta using spiralised vegetables is a fantastic replacement for heavy carbohydrate pasta. Courgette is my favourite, but you can use butternut squash, sweet potato, carrot or beetroot. It takes minutes to make. I don't have a big spiralising machine, because I prefer to keep my kitchen utensils to a minimum. Mine looks like a large pencil sharpener; it is easy to use and stores in my utensils drawer. Or you can use a vegetable peeler (see page 169).

Seeds

I have a range of seeds in containers in my cupboard. Flaxseeds, sesame seeds, pumpkin seeds and sunflower seeds are the ones I use every day. I often sauté some seeds in coconut oil and add these to my salads to give them a nice crunch and to add extra nutrients, or I use them to top my yogurt.

Chia seeds have a reputation as a superfood because they are packed with protein, omega-3 fatty acids, magnesium, manganese, phosphorus and a good source of fibre. They also contain vitamins B_1, B_2 and B_3 as well as iodine, iron, zinc and potassium. Chia seeds make a lovely creamy breakfast. They can also be used as a binder and vegan egg replacer.

Flaxseeds contain anti-inflammatory omega-3 fatty acids. They are also great for balancing the hormones due to the antioxidant lignans they contain. They provide protein and are good sources of manganese, vitamin B_1, magnesium and phosphorus, as well as B_6, folate, iron and zinc. I sprinkle flaxseeds on my yogurt as well as my salads. I also add them to my granola (page 93) and my savoury nut balls (page 207). Just like chia seeds, flaxseeds can be used as a binder and a vegan egg replacer.

Pumpkin seeds are known for their high zinc content, and are often recommended to men to help with prostate health. Pumpkin seeds also contain high levels of manganese, phosphorus, magnesium, copper and iron, and are packed with protein. They are good as a topping for yogurts and salads, and can also be used as snacks, especially when roasted.

Sunflower seeds are great to add as toppings for yogurts or salads. They also make good snacks and can be used to make a seed butter. They contain good sources of vitamin E, copper, B vitamins, magnesium, manganese, phosphorus and selenium.

Thickeners

Agar agar can be a direct replacement for gelatine, so it's ideal to use for desserts and jellies. Unlike gelatine, which is derived from animal bones, agar agar is suitable for vegans and vegetarians because it is made from an algae.

*

Arrowroot is a starch from the arrowroot plant. It is used in the same way that you would use cornflour, but it is grain-free.

Chia seeds are great to use to thicken mixtures and to make jams and are especially good as an egg binding replacement.

Cornflour can be used to thicken casseroles, soups, sauces and custards.

Flaxseeds are great to help thicken and bind mixtures.

Tomatoes

Tinned tomatoes You can always whip up a tasty dish if you have some tinned tomatoes. I always buy the best quality and organic, as I find the taste far nicer. You can also use passata, which is sieved tomatoes. This is good for sauces or soups where you need a smoother consistency.

Tomato purée is an essential to add flavour and depth to a dish. I also use sun-dried tomato paste, as I love the flavour. I often make this myself by whizzing up some sun-dried tomatoes in the food processor, but you can buy sugar-free sun-dried tomato paste in most supermarkets.

Yeast extract

Love it or hate it (I actually hate it), yeast extract it is very good to use in cooking for flavour as well as adding some essential vitamin B_{12} to your food. For those, like me, who dislike the taste, believe me, you can't taste it when it is added to savoury dishes.

Fridge essentials

Here are the fridge essentials that I wouldn't be without.

Butter/butter alternatives

Vegans don't eat butter, but if you are a part-time vegan, I would urge you to use butter and ditch any processed margarine and oils. Although you can buy vegan margarines, I don't recommend them, as they are processed fats and, as I have previously stated in this book, I only recommend the use of natural fats.

Coconut oil can be used as a butter alternative in cooking and works really well. You can also use coconut butter. (Read more about the uses for coconut oil on page 15.)

Alternatives If you want to spread a little butter or margarine on your bread but still want to be 100 per cent vegan, I would opt instead for nut butters (see page 67 for more details), mashed avocado, hummus or coconut oil. You can also dip your bread into some extra virgin olive oil.

Cream alternatives

There are a variety of dairy alternatives that can add a creamy texture to a dish or can even be suitable for puddings. Some are easy swaps – others take a little more preparation.

Cashew nuts When you soak cashew nuts for 1–2 hours, you can then process them to make a rich, creamy liquid or paste that can then be used in desserts, or added to soups or casseroles to give them a creamy consistency, or they can even be used as a replacement for ricotta or cottage cheese.

Coconut cream is one of my favourites for puddings and is great in curries. It is easy to get hold of and, unlike cashew nuts, needs no preparation. You can buy this in tins or cartons.

Coconut yogurt does tend to go a little thin when added to food, so it is not as good as coconut cream.

Silken tofu can be used to make creamy puddings.

Fruit

We are told to eat at least five portions of vegetables and fruit a day, and many people choose fruit to achieve this. Fruit is packed with antioxidants and vitamins, but it also contains a lot of fructose. I always advise people to opt for a diet richer in vegetables than fruit.

Berries are, for me, a must-have; they are not only tasty but they are also low in fructose and packed with antioxidants. I prefer raspberries and fresh blueberries. I buy frozen raspberries when the fresh berries not in season.

Lemon and limes I use a lot of lemons. I cut them into quarters and put them in the freezer to add to my drinks, as it doubles as an ice cube as well as adding a lemon flavour. I also use lemons in desserts and savouries for flavour.

Plant-based milk

There are a number of plant-based milks you can choose from. Always read the label, as some can contain added sugar or fruit concentrates to help sweeten them, and it is best to avoid these. All the milks, apart from soya milk, which is naturally higher in protein, fall short of essential nutrients such as vitamin B_{12}, calcium and protein content compared to dairy milk, which is why most plant-based milks are fortified with added nutrients to help boost their nutritional content.

Plant-based milks are much more expensive then dairy milk. Soya and almond milk are often the cheapest plant-based milks, but often these are non-organic varieties. Most plant-based milks contain only 2–10 per cent of the key ingredient – the main ingredient being water.

You can make your own nut milks, and it is surprisingly easy. If you feel like trying this, see the recipe on page 236.

Almond milk is much lower in protein than dairy milk and has to be fortified with added calcium and vitamins, such as B_2 and B_{12}, to boost the nutritional values. That said, the creamy, slightly nutty flavour is nice and mixes well in beverages.

Coconut milk is one of the most popular milks, along with all coconut products, but nutritionally it is a bit lacking. Like other plant-based milks, it has to be fortified with added calcium, B_{12} and vitamin D. It is very good in cooking, hot drinks and cereals.

Hemp milk is a good natural source of omega-3 and omega-6 fats. It is worth noting, however, for those who think that this is a good choice of omega-3, it is in the form of ALA (alpha linolenic acid) which is hard for the body to convert, so is not the same as type of omega-3 found in fish oil (see more on page 14). Hemp milk is low in protein. Most hemp milks are fortified with calcium and vitamin D and can have added thickeners in the ingredients. Hemp milk has a stronger flavour, which is more noticeable in beverages, but it is good in cooking.

*

Oat milk Like the majority of plant-based milks, oat milk is lower in protein and needs to be fortified with vitamins such as vitamins D, B_2 and B_{12}. Oats themselves are high in beta-glucan, which is great for heart health, but most plant milks contain mainly water with less than 10 per cent of the advertised ingredients, so if you are taking this to help reduce cholesterol and lower your blood pressure, you would be better getting your oats from other sources.

Rice milk is lower in protein than dairy milks and is fortified with calcium and vitamin B_{12}. It is often sweetened. I have found it quite watery compared to other plant milks. There has been some worrying reports that rice milk could contain traces of arsenic and the Food Standards Agency recommend it is not given to children under four.

Soya milk is the nearest in protein content to dairy milk, but it does have to be fortified to boost its calcium levels. The higher protein content can cause allergies similar to dairy allergies. There is quite a lot of concern regarding the health aspects of soya milk, including possible genetic modification and exposure to agrochemicals, which is why you should always opt for organic versions. Soya milk contains goitrogens, which can interfere with the uptake of iodine and, in turn, can lead to damage to the function of the thyroid. Soya also contains phytoestrogens, and there are a lot of mixed messages regarding this. Some phytoestrogens can have a negative effect on our health; for example, they can block our natural oestrogen function, increase the risk of cognitive decline and, in the case of breast cancer, could stimulate growth. I would advise you to avoid soya milk, as you can get much healthier food containing phytoestrogens. Soya milk doesn't work so well in beverages because it can curdle, but it is good for cooking. To summarise, given all the possible problems with soya milk, I would opt for one of the other plant-based milks.

You can also buy cashew milk and hazelnut milk.

Tofu and tempeh

Tofu, a traditional Japanese food, is a curd made from soya milk. Given the problems with soya listed above, I would opt only for organic tofu. It is a good product for vegans. You can make a great 'scrambled egg' with it, and it can be the base of a vegan quiche and some puddings. Tofu is quite tasteless, but it soaks up the flavour from other ingredients well. Tempeh, which originated in Indonesia, is made from fermented soya beans. It contains more protein than tofu and is a probiotic so it can aid gut health. It is also high in manganese. Just like tofu, tempeh absorbs flavours well so it can be added to most meals.

Yogurt

Dairy-free natural coconut yogurt is beautifully light. Be careful, however, as some varieties can contain added sugars and unnecessary additives.

Vegan 'cheat' meats

It'll come as no surprise to hear me say that I don't use vegan 'cheat' meats. I prefer real food, and if you're following this book as a part-time vegan, you can get your meat fix from the real thing, if needed. Real food, in my opinion, is always the best choice. If I want to emulate the taste and texture of meat, I opt to use natural foods. I have included a delicious vegan mince using mushrooms and walnuts (see page 191), which is far healthier and more natural than soya alternatives.

You could also use tofu, tempeh or vegetables, including jack-fruit, as meat substitutes.

Quorn has become quite popular, and I can understand its popularity, although I still prefer to eat real food. From what I have read, it is a better alternative to textured soya protein, but be careful, as it can cause some allergic reactions in those sensitive to proteins. Quorn contains MycoProtein, which is a processed product made from a fungus called *Fusarium venenatum*, produced using a fermentation process. You will need to check the label, as some Quorn products are made with egg, so not all of it is suitable for vegans. Quorn contains 10–15g of protein per 100g and has moderate carbs at approximately 4–10g per 100g, depending on the type of product you eat.

Textured soya protein (also called TVP) Some vegan meat products are made from rehydrated textured soya protein. It has gained popularity because it is cheap to produce and is claimed to be a good protein source for vegans. This is a very heavily processed pretend food and can contain some unsavoury additives and chemicals. Textured soya protein is a by-product of soybean oil, with the rather unattractive description of being a 'defatted soy flour product'. It does contain protein and some fibre, but that really is about it. Views are mixed in the vegan community, but I would definitely advise you to avoid it.

Vegan cheeses

You can now buy almost any style of cheese in vegan form. They have certainly improved over the years. Ingredients can vary and, as always, some are healthier than others. Check the ingredients list. If you can understand the ingredients, then go ahead and buy it, but if you need a chemistry degree, or if it is something your grandmother wouldn't see as food, avoid it! Personally, I don't like relying on these, as I prefer to eat the real thing in its natural form, but, for strict vegans, they can add variety to your meals.

Bought vegan cheese tends to have a base of starch and oils (mainly coconut oil) along with natural flavourings to create the texture and flavour of cheese.

Vegetables and salad

My weekly shop includes a huge percentage of vegetables. I choose a variety of vegetables, with the emphasis on seasonal veg where possible. I have recently signed up to an organic delivery scheme, as I was continually frustrated by my local supermarket stocking only a very small variety of organic vegetables. I'm enjoying the food that is delivered. It also makes my life easier and it is a joy to unpack a new box every week and discover the latest seasonal vegetable. I then spend half an hour or so planning my meals for the week ahead, ensuring I use up everything in the box. Anything left over either gets made into a soup or a meal and frozen.

I always have red onions, peppers, cauliflower, broccoli and sweet potatoes, with a wide range of green vegetables. I use celeriac a lot, as it is low carb and a great alternative to potato, especially to make celeriac chips (see page 151). I roast radishes and add them to casseroles, as they also are a tasty replacement for white potatoes. Mushrooms are versatile, especially when mixed with walnuts to create a vegan mince.

My fridge always contains lots of salad foods and avocados – a must have! Don't let your avocados go off, because you can freeze them (see page 61), and then use them in vegetable smoothies, guacamole and chocolate mousse.

Freezer Essentials

I have added the freezer here more for storing your own home-made ready meals. I am a huge fan of batch cooking, planning ahead and avoiding waste, and the freezer is an invaluable tool for that. We all lead busy lives, hence our passion for processed, quick-and-easy food. If we batch cook, by doubling up some recipes and freezing in individual or family portions, we are creating our own ready meals for days when we need to grab and go.

My youngest son has high-functioning autism. He absolutely adores cooking and has a real flair for it. He loves creating new dishes and cakes, but, like most teenagers, he also enjoys pizza. We make up our own pizza bases and store them in the freezer, ready for topping (see page 106 for recipe ideas).

Apart from all the homemade meals I store in the freezer, here are some of my other freezer essentials:

Frozen raspberries are always nice to have in the freezer for when you fancy a treat or just to have with some coconut yogurt and nuts.

Frozen vegetables I freeze my own vegetables. If something is not used up in time, I will dice it and freeze it. I chop my vegetables into useable chunks before putting them in freezer bags to freeze. I often do this with sweet potato, swede, parsnips, celeriac or carrots, which are ideal for adding to casseroles when I don't have any fresh veg to hand. Some people dislike frozen peas, but I love them. They are not the best vegetable nutritionally, but I add these to my steamed green veg. I also buy frozen broad beans, edamame beans and sweetcorn.

Herbs from the freezer

Fresh herbs are great, if you can grow them in pots or the garden. If you can't grow your own, or it is the wrong time of the year, try frozen herbs. You can buy freshly frozen herbs, which can last for months and offer a superior taste over dried varieties. If you grow your own and have a surplus, you can freeze herbs yourself. Herbs that freeze well are basil, coriander, oregano, sage, dill, rosemary, mint, lemongrass, chives, tarragon, and thyme. I also freeze fresh chillies, garlic and ginger. Use frozen herbs in cooking – they are not suitable for garnishes.

Ice cream I have included an ice cream recipe in the book (see page 221), but for store-bought ice creams, I opt for Oppo ice cream because it is sugar-free, but it isn't vegan; however, you can get a lot of vegan ice creams now, although some are very heavily processed, so check the ingredients list carefully. I would recommend looking at Booja-Booja, as their ice creams contain only five ingredients, and they are organic and low in sugar.

Part III

THE RECIPES

The following chapters feature recipes suitable for the whole family. All the recipes are vegan and most are gluten free, too. Some of the recipes, such as the lasagne, nut and mushroom balls, and bolognese are formulated to replicate their traditional meat counterpart, without the need for processed vegan meat alternatives. You'll also find a variety of sweet and savoury snack, all of which are sugar free.

Simple, Scrumptious Breakfasts

H ere, you will find no-hassle, quick-and-easy vegan breakfasts for people on the go. This chapter also includes some recipes that you might want to prepare in advance, such as my lovely granola recipe, which is far healthier than the processed, sugary alternatives from the supermarkets.

You can also adopt some of these easy, grab-and-dash ideas:

- Nut butter on buckwheat or spelt toast
- Nut butter on toast with grated apple topping
- Avocado on buckwheat or spelt toast
- Coconut yogurt with berries and nuts

Smoothies

Many people love the convenience of smoothies, especially with added protein powder to boost their protein levels. Smoothies are a great way to add essential nutrients while on the go. You can fill a smoothie with some healthy fats, such as avocado, chia seeds, flaxseeds or flax oils. You can also add some protein sources with activated (soaked) nuts, protein powders or soaked quinoa. Berries, in particular, are rich in antioxidants; however, a word of warning: try not to add too many high-fructose fruits to the smoothie or you may find your glass of innocent-looking smoothie contains more sugar than a glass of cola! If you are going to add fruit, opt for those with the least fructose, such as raspberries, strawberries and blueberries.

Avocado Smoothie

Avocados contain essential fatty acids, which fuel your body as well as helping to keep you feeling fuller for longer, so they are ideal for starting the day. They also add fantastic creaminess to a smoothie. Also included here are chia seeds for extra protein, and spinach for vitamin A, niacin, zinc and vitamin C.

Serves 1
  ½ avocado, flesh scooped from the skin
  30g baby leaf spinach
  2 tbsp coconut cream or non-dairy yogurt
  1 tsp chia seeds
  a small handful of blueberries
  100ml unsweetened almond milk or other plant-based milk,
    plus extra if needed

Put all the ingredients into a blender, food processor or Nutribullet and whizz until smooth. If you like a more liquid smoothie, add more milk to taste.

Nutritional information per serving: 118 kcal, 11g fat, 1.8g net carbohydrates, 2.1g protein

Chocolate Power Smoothie

Although I am not a huge fan of protein powders, they can be a great addition for those who are not getting enough protein in their diet. There are some good vegan protein powders available, but do check the ingredients and only buy the purest, unsweetened forms. This smoothie contains healthy fats and protein to keep you feeling full and satisfied.

Serves 1
- 250–350ml unsweetened almond milk or other
  plant-based milk
- 1 scoop of vegan, unsweetened protein powder
- 2 tsp cacao powder or unsweetened cocoa powder
- 1 tbsp coconut oil
- ½ avocado, flesh scooped from the skin
- 1 shot of espresso, cooled

Put 250ml of the milk into your blender, food processor or Nutribullet and add the remaining ingredients. Blend until smooth, adding more milk if needed to get the consistency you desire. Serve chilled.

Nutritional information per serving: 434 kcal, 32g fat, 4.3g net carbohydrates, 30g protein

Overnight Muesli

This recipe is the perfect grab-and-go-style breakfast that is easy to prepare and can be adapted to suit any flavour combination. If you like, you can make this in a jar or airtight container, ready to transport to work for breakfast the next day. It's full of healthy fats and protein from the almond butter, flaxseeds and chia seeds.

Serves 1
   150–200ml unsweetened almond milk or other
      plant-based milk
   3 tbsp oats
   1 tbsp chia seeds
   1 tbsp flaxseeds
   1 tbsp almond butter
   50g raspberries or blueberries

In the evening put 150ml of the milk in a jar or airtight container and add the remaining ingredients. Combine well, then leave overnight in the fridge.

Stir well before eating. You might want to add more milk to get the taste and texture you love.

Nutritional information per serving: 405 kcals, 24g fat, 24g net carbohydrates, 14g protein

Lemon and Blueberry Pancakes

This batter is best made in advance so that it's ready to cook in the morning. (It can be stored in an airtight container in the fridge for up to

24 hours.) Ensure you give it a good whisk before you start to fry the pancakes. If you are in a hurry, you can cook the pancakes in advance, then stack them between sheets of baking parchment until ready to reheat. When ready to eat, just pop them into the frying pan and heat them up. Alternatively, you can microwave them.

Makes 8 small pancakes

150g spelt or buckwheat flour

2 tsp baking powder

¼ tsp ground cinnamon

300ml unsweetened almond milk or other plant-based milk

1 tbsp coconut oil, melted, plus extra for frying

1 tsp vanilla extract

200g blueberries

juice from 1–2 lemons, to taste

a little xylitol or erythritol, or stevia drops to taste, or a drizzle
   of fibre syrup or rice malt syrup (optional)

Sift the flour, baking powder and cinnamon into a bowl. Put the milk, coconut oil and vanilla extract in a small bowl and mix well together.

Add this to the dry ingredients and combine well using a whisk. Leave for 30 minutes or overnight if possible.

Heat a little coconut oil in a frying pan over a medium heat. Pour a ladleful of the pancake batter into the pan, tilting the pan to cover the base.

Cook until golden on one side, then flip the pancake over and repeat on the other side until both sides of the pancake are golden.

Turn onto a plate, top with blueberries and a squeeze of lemon juice. If you like sweet pancakes, add a little sweetener.

Nutritional information per pancake:104 kcals, 2.5g fat, 15g net carbohydrates, 3.4g protein

Quinoa and Chia Porridge

Traditionally, quinoa porridge takes about 20 minutes to cook – so it's not a quick-and-easy workday breakfast! Soaking the mix overnight, plus using flaked quinoa, speeds up the whole process considerably, and so it is perfect if you love your nutritious porridge on a weekday. Serve it with some chopped nuts or a spoonful of nut butter and a handful of berries. In the winter months, I keep things simple and top with a sprinkle of Sukrin Gold, an erythritol blend, which tastes and looks just like brown sugar. This reminds me of my childhood when demerara sugar was my dad's favourite porridge topping.

Serves 1
  1 tbsp chia seeds
  30g flaked quinoa
  250ml unsweetened almond milk or other plant-based milk,
    plus extra if needed
  ½ tsp vanilla extract (optional)
  topping of choice, to serve

Put all the ingredients in a jar or an airtight container. Combine well, then cover with a lid and leave overnight in the fridge.

You can eat the porridge cold, but if you prefer it warm, tip the mixture into a saucepan. Heat over a medium heat, stirring continuously, until it starts to thicken. Continue cooking for 5 minutes or until it is heated through, adding more milk if needed, until you get the consistency you prefer.

Remove from the heat and top with your favourite topping before serving.

Nutritional information per serving: 178 kcals, 7.4g fat, 17g net carbohydrates, 8.2g protein

Chocolate, Goji and Coconut Granola

This is a store-cupboard essential for quick-and-easy breakfasts. It is really easy to make and there is nothing stopping you from doubling or tripling the quantities to make up a large batch, because it keeps well in a sealed, airtight container. I keep this in a large Kilner jar. As well as for breakfast, I eat this as a snack with yogurt, as a topping for desserts or to put in a bowl and munch in front of my favourite film!

Makes about 15 servings

300g mixed nuts (such as Brazil nuts, hazelnuts, almonds, macadamia nuts, walnuts)

100g pecan nuts (these add a sweetness that kids love)

75g flaked almonds

100g unsweetened coconut flakes

75g sunflower seeds

75g pumpkin seeds

40g coconut oil, melted (see tip below)

2 tbsp cacao powder or unsweetened cocoa powder

2 tbsp xylitol or erythritol blend, or to taste

80g oats

60g goji berries

Preheat the oven to 150°C (130°C fan oven) Gas 2. Put the mixed nuts and pecan nuts in a freezer bag and bash them with a rolling pin until they are in smaller pieces. (I prefer doing it this way, as it takes out my frustrations, and although you can use a food processor it tends to overprocess the nuts and, if you are not careful, you can end up with nutty dust!)

Put the crushed nuts in a bowl and add the flaked almonds, half the coconut flakes and all the seeds.

Heat the oil in a jug (see tip), and add the cacao and sweetener, then combine well.

Pour over the nut mix and stir until well coated.

Pour the nut mixture onto a large baking tray – you might need 2 trays depending on the size of your tray. Spread it out evenly until it covers the tray.

Pop into the oven and bake for 5 minutes, then turn the nuts and bake for another 5 minutes. Remove from the oven and cool, then stir in the remaining coconut flakes with the oats and goji berries. Store in an airtight container for up to 2 weeks.

Nutritional information per serving: 347 kcals, 32g fat, 4g net carbo-hydrates, 8.2g protein

To melt coconut oil: I melt my coconut oil in the microwave, but you can also melt it in a saucepan on a low/medium heat or place the coconut oil in a bowl and place this in a larger bowl of hot water.

Cinnamon and Apple Granola

This is really great as a breakfast granola and also as a topping for fruit crumbles, added to coconut yogurt or just as a tasty snack.

Makes about 15 servings

    300g mixed nuts (such as Brazil nuts, hazelnuts, almonds, macadamia nuts, walnuts)

    100g pecan nuts

    60g flaked almonds

    100g coconut flakes

    75g sunflower seeds

    75g pumpkin seeds

    50g flaxseeds

    40g coconut oil, melted

2 tsp ground cinnamon

½ tsp ground mixed spice

½ tsp allspice

2 tbsp xylitol or erythritol blend, or to taste

80g oats

75g dried apple slices, halved

Preheat the oven to 150°C (130°C fan oven) Gas 2. Put the nuts in a freezer bag and bash with a rolling pin until they are in smaller pieces. (Although you can use a food processor it tends to overprocess the nuts and you can end up with nutty dust!)

Put the crushed nuts in a bowl and add the flaked almonds, coconut flakes and seeds.

Put the coconut oil in a jug, and add the spices and sweetener, then combine well.

Pour over the nut mix and stir well until the oil coats all the nuts.

Pour the nut mixture onto a large baking tray – you might need 2 trays depending on the size of your tray. Spread it out until it covers the tray.

Pop into the oven and bake for 5 minutes, then turn the nuts and bake for another 5 minutes.

Remove from the oven and cool, then stir in the oats and dried apple slices. Store in an airtight container for up to 2 weeks.

Nutritional information per serving: 375 kcals, 32g fat, 9.5g net carbohydrates, 9.4g protein

Basic Chia Porridge

Chia seeds are packed full of protein. I use them a lot in cooking. They absorb liquid, so they are a great thickener. This recipe is for a basic chia porridge to which you can add fruit, a spoonful of cacao or cocoa, a mashed banana or shredded coconut. Top with whatever takes your fancy.

This needs to be prepared at least an hour in advance, but ideally the night before.

Serves 2
    250ml unsweetened almond milk or other plant-based milk,
        plus extra if needed
    60g chia seeds
    1 tsp of vanilla extract (optional)
    a sprinkle of xylitol or erythritol, or stevia drops, to taste
    nuts and berries, to serve

Put the milk and chia seeds in a bowl or jug, then stir in the vanilla extract. Leave to rest in the fridge for an hour or overnight.

You can eat this hot or cold, but if you prefer it warm, tip the mixture into a saucepan. Heat over a low heat until it is heated through, adding more milk if needed.

Finish with a sprinkle of natural sweetener and some nuts and berries.

Nutritional information per serving: 219 kcals, 13.9g fat, 7.8g net carbohydrates, 9.6g protein

Variation: This is also delicious mixed with some nut butter. Add 2 tablespoons to the chia seeds and milk before leaving the mixture to soak.

Weekend and Slouch-Day Breakfasts

These recipes are perfect for a lazy morning brunch when you have time to kick back, chill out, read the papers and enjoy your coffee in peace, while you wait for your leisurely breakfast or brunch. Even better, why not get someone else to make your breakfast for you? Failing that, scan through the pages in this chapter, as some can be prepped the day or evening before and stored in the fridge.

Vegetable Kedgeree

This is such a versatile dish it was hard to decide where to put it in the book! It can be a great breakfast or brunch for the weekend or it can be served as a main meal. You can use any leftovers for a delicious cold rice salad or can even to accompany a curry.

You can also make this using cauliflower rice (see page 72), which is great if you want to reduce your carb intake.

Serves 4

    2 tsp coconut oil or olive oil
    1 red onion

1 garlic clove, crushed

3 cardamom pods, crushed

¼–½ tsp chilli flakes, to taste (optional)

½ tsp ground turmeric

½ tsp ground coriander

1 tsp paprika

300g brown basmati rice

1 litre vegetable stock, plus extra if needed

150g asparagus

1 head of broccoli, cut into florets

100g baby leaf spinach

Heat the oil in a saucepan over a medium heat and cook the onion, garlic and spices for 5 minutes, stirring frequently. Add the rice and vegetable stock. Bring to the boil, then reduce the heat and simmer for 5 minutes.

Snap off the coarse ends of the asparagus and discard them, then cut the spears into short pieces. Add the broccoli to the pan and cook for 8 minutes or until the rice and broccoli are cooked and the liquid has almost dispersed. Add a little more stock if the rice begins to dry out.

Add the asparagus and spinach, and stir well. Add a little more stock, if needed, stirring well. Cook over a low heat for 5 minutes or until tender. Season with salt and pepper to taste and serve hot or cold.

Nutritional information per serving: 390 kcals, 6.1g fat, 68g net carbohydrates, 11g protein

Scrambled Tofu with Roasted Garlic and Thyme Tomatoes

The thyme tomatoes in this simple recipe add a delicious flavour to the mild tofu. They are also a useful way to make a quick and delicious pasta sauce – just whizz them up in a blender or food processor. Nutritional yeast flakes give the tofu a lovely cheese flavour.

Serves 2

    1–2 tsp coconut oil, melted, or olive oil, plus extra for greasing

    3 tomatoes, halved

    1–2 garlic cloves, to taste, roughly chopped

    leaves from a few thyme sprigs

    ground black pepper

    slices of avocado, to serve (optional)

For the scrambled tofu:

    2 tsp coconut oil or olive oil

    400g block organic tofu, crumbled

    3 tbsp unsweetened almond milk or other plant-based milk, plus extra if needed

    2 tbsp nutritional yeast flakes

    black pepper

Preheat the grill and grease a baking tray. Put the tomatoes, cut side up, on the baking tray. Put the garlic and thyme on top of each of the tomatoes, then season with black pepper. Finish with a drizzle of coconut oil.

Cook under the grill until the tomatoes start to soften.

Meanwhile, to make the scrambled tofu, put the coconut oil in a saucepan over a medium heat and add the tofu. Stir in the milk. As the tofu gets hot it should become more pliable. Stir until the tofu looks like scrambled eggs to the consistency you like (add more milk if you like a runnier mix).

Add the nutritional yeast flakes and season with black pepper. Serve with the grilled tomatoes and slices of avocado, if you like.

Nutritional information per serving: 465 kcals, 26g fat, 13g net carbohydrates, 39g protein

Smoky Baked Beans

I have popped this recipe into the breakfast chapter, but it can also make a quick-and-easy lunch. These smoky baked beans can be frozen, so you can save time and double up the recipe and freeze in individual portions. Serve on top of your favourite toasted bread.

■ Double up and freeze

Serves 6
   ½ tsp coconut oil or olive oil
   1 red onion, diced
   2 garlic cloves, roughly chopped
   2 × 400g tins haricot or cannellini beans, drained and rinsed
   500g passata
   2 tbsp sun-dried tomato paste or tomato purée
   a dash of vegan Worcestershire sauce or coconut aminos
   1 tsp wholegrain mustard
   ½ tsp ground cumin
   ½ tsp chilli powder
   1–2 tsp smoked paprika, to taste (optional)
   ground black pepper to taste

Put the oil in a saucepan over a medium-low heat and cook the onion and garlic for 5 minutes or until it starts to soften. Add the remaining ingredients and combine well. Bring to the boil, then reduce the heat and simmer gently for 10 minutes.

   Store any leftovers in the fridge for up to 1 week or freeze.

Nutritional information per 100g serving: 92 kcals, 1.9g fat, 11g net carbohydrates, 4.4g protein

Vegan Shakshouka

Here is an adaptation of the Middle Eastern dish of the same name, which is traditionally made with poached eggs. It's simple to make and I like to pop it in the oven while I get ready for the day. You can add some grilled tofu to the dish if you like, although I don't think it needs anything.

Serves 2

    1 tsp coconut oil or olive oil

    1 small red onion, sliced

    1–2 garlic cloves, to taste, roughly chopped

    1 red or yellow pepper, deseeded and sliced

    ½ courgette, sliced

    60g chestnut mushrooms, quartered

    400g tin chopped tomatoes

    1 tsp paprika

    2 tsp fresh or 1 tsp dried oregano

    1 sprig of fresh or ½ tsp dried thyme

    1 tsp ground cumin

    a small handful of fresh parsley leaves, chopped

    ½ tsp chilli powder (optional)

    crusty buckwheat, spelt or low carb, grain-free bread, to serve

Heat the oil in a saucepan over a medium heat and cook the onion, garlic, pepper, courgette and mushrooms for 2 minutes to soften.

Add the remaining ingredients, except the bread, and bring to the boil, then reduce the heat and simmer gently for 10 minutes. Serve with crusty bread.

Nutritional information per serving: 152 kcals, 3.2g fat, 19g net carbohydrates, 6.2g protein

Hash Brown Stack

There is a lovely contrast of textures in this dish with the slightly crispy hash browns and the creamy avocados. It's a good idea to make these hash browns in advance and freeze them (either raw or cooked), ready to pop into the oven when you want them. The avocados provide plenty of healthy fat and the dish is also rich in vitamins.

Serves 4
  2 sweet potatoes, grated
  1 carrot, grated
  1 red onion, finely chopped
  2 garlic cloves, finely chopped
  2 tbsp fine polenta
  2 tbsp nutritional yeast flakes
  1 tsp paprika
  1 tbsp melted coconut or olive oil
  salt and ground black pepper

To serve:
  2 avocados, flesh scooped from the skin and sliced
  3 tomatoes, sliced
  1–2 tbsp balsamic vinegar, to taste
  2 tbsp olive oil

Preheat the oven to 180°C (160°C fan oven) Gas 4 and line a baking sheet with baking parchment. Put the grated potatoes in a tea towel and squeeze out as much moisture as you possibly can.

Put the potato in a bowl and add the remaining ingredients. Combine well and season with salt and pepper to taste.

Divide the mixture into 8 portions. Using your hands flatten one portion into a disc about 2cm thick. Put it onto the prepared baking sheet. Repeat with the remaining mixture to make 8 hash browns.

Cook in the oven for 30 minutes, or until golden. To create the stack, put a hash brown onto the plate. Add some slices of avocado, followed by some slices of tomatoes. Finish with another hash brown, then drizzle with balsamic vinegar and olive oil

Nutritional information per serving 410 kcals, 22g fat, 40g net carbo-hydrates, 7.6g protein

Mushrooms on Spelt Toast

Make this for a lazy Sunday morning brunch. You can use any variety of mushrooms. I like a mixture of oyster, shiitake, chestnut and baby mushrooms. If you're not vegan you can use butter instead of the olive oil, if you prefer, to give this a rich flavour.

Serves 2

   1 tsp coconut oil or olive oil
   1 tbsp olive oil
   2 garlic cloves, finely chopped
   75g chestnut mushrooms, quartered
   75g baby mushrooms
   50g baby leaf spinach
   a small handful of parsley leaves, chopped
   2 tsp thyme leaves or ½ tsp dried thyme
   juice of ¼ lemon (optional)
   4 slices of spelt bread
   2 tbsp homemade hummus (see page 141)
   seasoning to taste

Heat the coconut and olive oil in a saucepan and over a medium heat and cook the garlic and mushrooms for 5 minutes or until they start to soften.

Add the spinach, parsley and thyme – you might need to do this a little at a time, as it can take time for the spinach to wilt, but persevere and keep stirring the spinach in – it will disappear into almost nothing eventually!

Add the lemon juice and season. Toast the bread, then spread it with the hummus. Put the mushroom mixture on top, and serve.

Nutritional information per serving: 488 kcals, 14g fat, 64g net carbohydrates, 21g protein

Work-Day Lunches

Work lunches can be monotonous and dull, so why not liven things up by planning ahead? You can turn your leftover dinners into wonderful lunches and use your freezer to double up meals and create individual portions ready to be reheated in the office. If you don't have any facilities to reheat food, opt for delicious salads in the summer months and then, when it starts to chill off, fill a flask with soups and casseroles.

I've included lots of salads; all are suitable for workday lunches and all can be prepared in advance. I would also recommend the dips: hummus, guacamole and salsa can make a delicious and surprisingly nutritious lunch when combined with vegetable sticks, thick slices of cucumber or wraps. You can also add nut butter, but do ensure it only contains nuts and no other ingredients such as palm oil and sugars. You will find an easy recipe for nut butter in the Everyday Basic Recipes chapter. I can quite happily munch away on vegetable sticks, dips, nut butter and a handful of fresh cherry tomatoes.

Buckwheat Pizza

You can make pizza bases with vegetables such as broccoli or cau-liflower, which are delicious, but I find that they crumble if you don't add an egg to the base. This is a buckwheat base, so it's a healthier version than the standard wheat bases we are all used to. I have added my favourite topping, but you can adapt whatever suits your taste. If you want to add some extra protein try garlicky butter beans or slices of tempeh or tofu.

■ Get ahead – this dish can be prepared in advance

Makes 8 slices
    175g buckwheat flour, plus extra for dusting
    ½ tsp baking powder
    ¼ tsp chilli powder (optional)
    20g chia seeds
    ½ tsp dried Italian herbs

For the topping:
    3 tbsp sun-dried tomato paste
    1 small red onion, finely chopped
    ½ red pepper, deseeded and sliced
    40g chestnut mushrooms, sliced
    40g stoneless black Kalamata olives, halved
    60g rocket
    olive oil, for drizzling

Sift the buckwheat flour, baking powder and chilli powder, if using, into a bowl. Add the chia seeds and herbs. Stir to combine well.

Add 200ml water, a little at a time, and stir well using a fork to form a dough. Leave for 5 minutes, then use your hands to form the dough into a ball. You may need to add a little more water if it is too dry. Preheat the oven to 180°C (160°C fan oven) Gas 4, or your standard pizza setting.

Knead the dough on a lightly floured work surface for a good 5 minutes. Add a little more flour if it is too sticky, or a little more water if it is too dry.

Roll it out gently to form circle about 22cm in diameter and put it onto a baking sheet.

If, like me, you prefer a well-cooked dough, cook for 10 minutes then add the toppings. Otherwise, add the toppings first.

Spread the sun-dried tomato paste over the pizza base, then top with the onion, pepper, mushrooms and olives. Cook in the oven for a further 10 minutes if the base has been precooked, otherwise cook for 20 minutes.

Put the rocket on top of the hot pizza. Drizzle with some olive oil and serve immediately.

Nutritional information per slice: 191 kcals, 9.4g fat, 19g net carbohydrates, 4.5g protein

Get ahead: The dough can be made in advance and kept in the fridge for up to 24 hours. Alternatively, you can freeze the rolled-out pizza bases between sheets of baking parchment to prevent them sticking together.

Thai Bean Cakes

Serve these cakes with an interesting salad for a tasty working lunch. You can dip the cakes into some sweet chilli sauce, if you like. If you don't have cannellini beans in the store-cupboard you can also use chickpeas. I have even made the same recipe with mashed sweet potato (into a sort of Thai potato cake) and it has worked well.

Serves 4

  400g tin cannellini beans, drained and rinsed
  ½ bunch of spring onions, finely chopped
  a handful of coriander leaves, finely chopped
  1 tbsp red Thai paste
  zest of 1 lime
  juice of ½ lime
  flour, for dusting
  2 tsp coconut oil

Shake the drained beans dry. Put them in a food processor and add the onions, coriander, Thai paste, and the lime zest and juice, then and whizz until combined.

  Put the mixture onto a floured work surface and form into 4 cakes.

  Heat the oil in frying pan and cook the bean cakes on both sides for 8–10 minutes or until golden. Serve. The cakes can be stored in the fridge for up to 3 days or frozen.

Nutritional information per serving: 140 kcals, 5.3g fat, 15g net carbohydrates, 6g protein

Spicy Sweet Potato and Chickpea Balls

These are very similar to falafels and are perfect with a salad. They can be prepared in advance and will store in the fridge for up to 5 days. I line the container with some kitchen paper to keep them dry. The recipe uses 1 chilli, but if you prefer a bit more of a kick, double this.

Serves 4

  2 sweet potatoes, cut into cubes
  400g tin chickpeas, drained and rinsed

unsweetened almond milk or other plant-based milk, if needed

1 tsp coconut oil or olive oil

1 red onion chopped

1–2 garlic cloves, to taste, crushed

1 chilli, deseeded and finely chopped

1 tsp ground turmeric

2 tsp paprika

½–2 tsp chilli powder, to taste

¼ tsp cayenne pepper

4 tbsp fine polenta

salt and ground black pepper

mixed salad, to serve

Preheat the oven to 180°C (160°C fan oven) Gas 4. Put the sweet potatoes in a steamer and steam over a high heat for 5–8 minutes until tender. Put the sweet potatoes in a bowl and add the chickpeas. Mash well, adding a little milk if needed. Leave to one side.

Melt the coconut oil in a saucepan and fry the onion, garlic and chilli for 5 minutes or until tender. Add the spices and stir for 1 minute.

Remove from the heat and add this mixture to the mash. Mix well and season to taste.

Take a small amount of the mash in your hands and form into small balls the size of golf balls.

Put the polenta on a plate and roll the balls individually in the polenta to give them a crisp coating. Put on a baking tray and cook in the oven for 15–20 minutes. Serve with a mixed salad.

Nutritional information per serving: 266 kcals, 5g fat, 44g net carbohydrates, 7.5g protein

Tofu and Spinach Quiche

This quiche is one of my favourites, and it is a big hit with meat eaters, as well as vegetarians and vegans – most people don't realise they are eating tofu! It keeps well in the fridge, so it could last you a few days. As always, use organic tofu. The fat content of this recipe is due to the coconut oil, so it's from a healthy fat. If you like, you can double up the quantities and freeze one quiche.

■ Double up and freeze

Serves 8

250g spelt or buckwheat flour, plus extra for dusting
125g coconut oil, chilled and cut into small pieces, plus extra
   for greasing
400g organic tofu
unsweetened almond milk or other plant-based milk, if needed
80g baby leaf spinach
50g nutritional yeast flakes
1 onion, finely chopped
a dash of finely grated nutmeg
seasoning

Put the flour in a food processor and add the coconut oil. Whizz until the mix resembles breadcrumbs. (Alternatively, rub the coconut oil gently into the flour using your fingers, but try not to handle the mixture too much.)

Add 2–4 tbsp cold water, a little at a time, and mix with a fork until it comes together. Use your hands to form a dough. Wrap the dough in cling film and put it in the fridge to rest for 30 minutes or until needed.

Preheat the oven to 200°C (180°C fan oven) Gas 6 and grease a 23cm flan tin. Roll out the pastry on a lightly floured work surface to a bit larger than the tin and line the tin.

Put a sheet of baking parchment over the pastry and cover it with baking beans. Bake for 10 minutes. Remove the baking beans and parchment, and cook for a further 10 minutes until the pastry starts to colour. Remove the pastry case from the oven and reduce the heat to 180°C (160°C fan oven) Gas 4.

While the pastry is baking, mash the tofu thoroughly – you can add some milk to help, if needed.

Put the spinach in a colander and rinse well with hot water from the kettle until it starts to wilt. Stir into the tofu.

Add the nutritional yeast flakes, the onion and nutmeg. If the mixture is too dry, add a dash of milk and mix well. Season then pour the mixture into the pastry case.

Bake for 20 minutes or until golden.

Nutritional information per serving: 326 kcals, 19g fat, 23g net carbohydrates, 12g protein

The Smart Sandwich

I am not a fan of wheat bread, so I've suggested using bread made with the traditional grains spelt or buckwheat. If those don't appeal to you, opt for something as unprocessed as possible, such as a simple brown sourdough. This sandwich is packed with healthy fats from the guacamole and a good range of protein and complex carbohydrates from the chickpeas and the bread – ideal for slow energy release, and perfect to fill you up.

Serves 1
   2 slices of spelt or buckwheat bread
   1 tbsp homemade hummus (see page 141)
   1 tbsp homemade guacamole (see page 143)

a few mixed salad leaves
2 thin slices of red pepper
1 small tomato, sliced
4 slices of cucumber
salt and ground black pepper

Spread one slice of bread with hummus and the other slice with the guacamole.

Put the mixed leaves, pepper, slices of tomato and cucumber on top of one slice.

Season with salt and pepper to taste, then pop on the top slice. Cut in half and wrap in baking parchment to store until lunchtime.

Nutritional information per serving: 533 kcals, 19g fat, 65g net carbohydrates, 18g protein

Minted Vegetable and Chickpea Quinoa

I love the combination of the fresh vegetables and chickpeas with the refreshing flavour of mint. If taking this to work, you might want to put the dressing in a separate container and add it just before you eat. It won't hurt to add it in the morning, but the dish does seem to keep better without.

Serves 4
    120g quinoa
    ½ tsp ground turmeric
    50g peas
    50g sweetcorn frozen, or tinned, drained and rinsed
    4 spring onions, finely chopped
    1 red pepper, deseeded and diced
    2 tomatoes, diced

¼ cucumber, diced
50g sugar snap peas, diced
1 celery stick, diced
400g tin chickpeas, drained and rinsed
2 tsp finely chopped mint leaves
seasoning to taste

For the dressing:
4 tbsp olive oil
juice of 1 lemon

Put the quinoa and turmeric in a saucepan and add 300ml water. Bring to the boil then reduce the heat and cook for 5 minutes. Now add the peas and sweetcorn, bring back to the boil and cook for another 5–10 minutes. Keep an eye on the water level: it should evaporate slowly but not enough to make the quinoa burn. Add more water if needed.

Drain the quinoa and add the remaining ingredients. Combine well and season with salt and pepper to taste.

To make the dressing, mix the olive oil with the lemon juice and season to taste.

When ready to serve, pour the dressing over the quinoa and combine well. This can be prepared in advance and will keep well in the fridge, stored in an airtight container, for up to 3 days, as long as you don't add any dressing until ready to eat.

Nutritional information per serving with dressing: 342 kcals, 17g fat, 32g net carbohydrates, 11g protein

Soups

I am a huge fan of soups. They can make wonderful and nutritious lunches with the added advantage of being cheap and filling – and you can pop them in a flask. A soup is also a great way to add more vegetables to your diet as well as using up any spare vegetables you have in your fridge. Most of the recipes that follow can be frozen, so consider doubling them up so that you have your own ready meals to hand when you have a frantic day.

Soup-making tips

- **Stock** I don't use stock cubes, as I find them far too salty and they totally overpower the natural flavours. I make a vegetable stock (see page 244), to allow the ingredients to speak for themselves.
- **Puréeing soups** Some people like a chunky soup, others like a smooth soup. It is purely personal taste. When puréeing a soup, I use an electric stick blender. It is simple to use (although make sure the end of the blender is fully submerged in the soup or you will end up with it everywhere). For a really fine soup, you can filter it through a sieve.
- **Slow cooker** I make my soups in a slow cooker unless I am in a hurry and have forgotten to prepare something earlier. The beauty of slow cooking is that it retains the food's nutrients. If you don't have a slow cooker, try to get into the habit of cooking slowly over low heats to help preserve the nutrients.
- **Chunky soups** Some chunky soups may benefit from a thicker base. To do this, simply remove about a quarter of the soup and purée it using a blender, then return it to the soup.

- **Coconut milk/cream** I use coconut cream or creamed coconut to make a creamy soup. Creamed coconut is bought in blocks and you have to pop it into a jar of hot water to soften it. Alternatively, you can buy a carton of coconut cream or use the cream from a tin of coconut milk. If you are using a tin, see page 64 for advice on how to scoop off the cream easily.
- **Nut butters** Adding a tablespoon or two of nut butters or tahini can give a nice richness to a soup as well as adding to the protein and fat content.

Butternut Squash Soup

Serve this filling and comforting soup in autumn when there is a lovely variety of squashes – but it's also great at any time of the year. You can play about with the spices to suit your palate – here it has a kick of chilli and a drizzle of chilli oil on top to serve.

■ Double up and freeze

Serves 4

1 tsp coconut oil or olive oil

1 red onion, diced

1–2 garlic cloves, to taste, crushed

1 tsp coriander seeds

300g butternut squash, peeled, deseeded and diced

1 tsp ground coriander

1 tsp paprika

½ tsp chilli flakes (optional)

1 small cooking apple, cored and diced

450ml vegetable stock, plus extra if needed

seasoning to taste

a drizzle of chilli oil (optional), to serve

Heat the oil in a saucepan over a medium heat and cook the onion, garlic and coriander seeds for 3–4 minutes until softened.

Add the butternut squash, coriander, paprika and chilli flakes, if using, and cook for 4 minutes, stirring regularly.

Add the apple and the stock. Bring to the boil, then reduce the heat to medium-low. Cover with a lid and cook for 20 minutes or until tender.

Season to taste, then purée using a blender or food processor. You can add more stock if you prefer a more liquid soup. Return the soup to the pan and reheat. Serve the soup with a drizzle of chilli oil in the centre, if you like.

Nutritional information per serving: 102 kcals, 2.9g fat, 15g net carbohydrates, 2g protein

Winter Vegetable, Quinoa and Lentil Soup

This is a chunky soup, so cut all your vegetables into even bite-sized pieces, to ensure they cook evenly. This makes eight portions, so freeze any leftovers. Although you could make a smaller quantity, it would mean halving lots of the vegetables and that could lead to waste.

■ Double up and freeze

Serves 8

1 tsp coconut oil or olive oil

2 garlic cloves, finely chopped

1 red onion, finely chopped

1 red pepper, deseeded and diced

1 carrot, diced

2 celery sticks, diced

1 small sweet potato, diced

1 leek, finely chopped

1 small parsnip, diced

100g quinoa, rinsed

1 litre vegetable stock, plus extra if needed

400g tin chopped tomatoes

2 tbsp sun-dried tomato paste

1 tsp paprika

1 bay leaf

50g red lentils

1 tbsp chopped parsley leaves or 1 tsp dried parsley

seasoning to taste

60g baby leaf spinach

Heat the oil in a large saucepan over a medium heat and cook the garlic and vegetables for 5 minutes. Add the quinoa to the vegetables, then add the remaining ingredients except the spinach.

Bring to the boil, then reduce the heat and simmer for 35 minutes, stirring occasionally, or until all the vegetables are cooked. You may need to add more stock while it is cooking.

Five minutes before serving, add the spinach. Stir in well to allow it to wilt and submerge into the soup. Continue to cook for 5 minutes, then serve.

Nutritional information per serving: 204 kcals, 7g fat, 26g net carbohydrates, 6g protein

Creamy Spinach, Kale and Broccoli Soup

My son calls this our green soup. It is a vibrant, creamy soup, packed with nutrients and healthy fats. You can use cavolo nero, also known as black kale, when it is in season.

■ Double up and freeze

Serves 6

2 tsp coconut oil or olive oil
1 onion, diced
1 garlic clove, crushed
1 celery stick, diced
400g tin coconut milk
400ml vegetable stock, plus extra if needed
1 head of broccoli, broken into small florets
80g kale, roughly chopped
80g baby leaf spinach
2 tsp finely chopped mint leaves or 1 tsp dried mint
seasoning to taste
1 avocado, flesh scooped from the skin and chopped
juice of 1 lime
mint leaves, to garnish

Heat the oil in a large saucepan over a medium heat and cook the onion, garlic and celery for 1 minute. Add the coconut milk and stock.

Add the broccoli, kale and spinach. (As this might overpower the saucepan until they start to heat through and soften, you can add them gradually if it helps.) Allow the spinach and kale to soften and reduce into the pan.

Add the mint and season to taste – I find it is best with a generous seasoning of black pepper. Cook for 20 minutes, then add the avocado and the lime juice.

Purée using a blender or food processor, adding more vegetable stock if needed until you reach your desired consistency. Return the soup to the pan and reheat. Serve garnished with mint.

Nutritional information per serving: 223 kcals, 19g fat, 7.4g net carbohydrates, 4.2g protein

Variation: As an option, you could omit the mint and add a handful of coriander leaves, chopped, ½ tsp chilli flakes and ½ tsp ground cumin.

Red Pepper and Tomato Soup with a Pesto Swirl

Homemade pesto is a wonderful topping for this rich and vibrant tomato and pepper soup.

■ Double up and freeze

Serves 6
    5 tomatoes
    1 tsp coconut oil or olive oil
    1 red onion, chopped
    1–2 garlic cloves, to taste
    2 red peppers, deseeded and diced
    ½ tsp mild chilli powder
    1 tsp paprika
    2 tbsp sun-dried tomato paste
    500ml vegetable stock

seasoning to taste

4 tsp Sun-dried Tomato Pesto (see page 239)

Plunge the tomatoes into boiling water for 30 seconds, then refresh in cold water. Peel away the skins. Chop and leave to one side.

Heat the oil in a large saucepan over a medium heat and cook the onion, garlic and peppers for 5–10 minutes until they start to soften and the onions are translucent. Add the chilli powder and paprika, and stir well to combine.

Add the tomatoes, tomato paste and stock, and season to taste. Cook over a medium-low heat for 20 minutes. Cool slightly, then purée using a blender or food processor. Return the soup to the pan and reheat. Serve the soup with a spoonful of homemade vegan pesto in the centre.

Nutritional information per serving: 154 kcals, 9.5g fat, 11g net carbohydrates, 3g protein

Variation: You can also make this soup with roasted peppers. Put the peppers on a baking tray under the grill and add a dash of balsamic vinegar. Grill, turning, until charred all over. Remove from the heat and cover the peppers with an upturned heatproof bowl. Leave to cool, then peel off the skins. Use the peppers in the soup.

Mint and Green Pea Soup

Fresh mint gives pea soup a fantastic flavour, so don't be tempted to use dried mint – it really won't be the same.

■ Double up and freeze

Serves 4

  1 tsp coconut oil or olive oil
  6 spring onions, chopped
  500ml vegetable stock
  500g peas (fresh or frozen)
  leaves from 3 mint sprigs, plus extra sprigs to garnish
  3 tbsp coconut cream
  black pepper to taste

Heat the oil in a large saucepan over a medium heat and cook the spring onions for 2 minutes. Add the stock, peas and mint, and season with black pepper. Cook gently over a low heat for 15 minutes.

Cool slightly, then purée using a blender or food processor. Return the soup to the pan and reheat. Stir in the coconut cream and adjust the seasoning to taste.

Serve hot, with a mint sprig to garnish. (Alternatively, you can leave the soup to cool, then put it in the fridge to serve chilled.)

Nutritional information per serving: 185 kcals, 6.9g fat, 17g net carbohydrates, 10g protein

Minestrone Soup

This is a very filling and delicious soup, perfect for a satisfying lunch. I don't add pasta to my minestrone soup, so a bit of artistic licence is needed. When you chop the vegetables, ensure that they are equal bite-sized pieces – it makes such a difference. If you don't want to use fresh tomatoes, you can swap them for a 400g tin chopped tomatoes.

▨ Double up and freeze

Serves 6

 4 tomatoes

 1 tsp coconut oil or olive oil

 1 red onion, chopped

 2 garlic cloves, crushed

 1 red pepper, deseeded and finely chopped

 1 carrot, finely diced

 ½ celery stick, finely chopped

 400g tin cannellini or haricot beans, drained and rinsed

 500ml vegetable stock

 1 tbsp sun-dried tomato paste

 3 tsp fresh oregano or 2 tsp dried oregano

 2 tsp thyme leaves or ½ tsp dried thyme

 1 tsp paprika

 2 bay leaves

 50g green beans, chopped

 50g cabbage, finely shredded

 50g baby leaf spinach

 seasoning to taste

Plunge the tomatoes into boiling water for 30 seconds, then refresh in cold water. Peel away the skins, then chop the flesh. Leave to one side.

Heat the oil in a large saucepan over a medium heat and cook the onion and garlic for 2 minutes. Add pepper and cook for another 2 minutes.

Add the remaining ingredients, except for the green beans, cabbage and spinach, and cook over a low heat for 25 minutes.

Add the green beans, cabbage and spinach, season and cook for another 10 minutes.

Nutritional information per serving 150 kcals, 4.5g fat, 18g net carbo-hydrates, 5.5g protein

Roasted Pumpkin Soup

Although this recipe uses pumpkin, it will work well with any squash. It has a fantastic flavour and sweetness due to the roasting beforehand. If you want to be fancy, you could serve the soup inside small hollowed-out roasted pumpkins – a wonderful way to celebrate Hallowe'en.

▨ Double up and freeze

Serves 6

- 1 small pumpkin, unpeeled, cut into wedges and deseeded
- 1 tsp coconut oil or olive oil, plus 1 tsp coconut oil, melted, or olive oil, for brushing the pumpkin
- 4 tomatoes
- 1 red onion, chopped
- 2 garlic cloves, crushed
- 2cm piece of fresh ginger, peeled and grated
- 1 tsp finely grated nutmeg
- 1 tsp ground coriander
- 2 carrots, chopped
- 1 sweet potato, chopped
- 2 celery sticks, chopped
- 1 tbsp tomato purée
- 500ml vegetable stock
- 15ml lemon juice
- seasoning to taste

Preheat the oven to 160°C (140°C fan oven) Gas 2½. Brush the pumpkin with a light coating of coconut oil and roast it for 20 minutes. Meanwhile, plunge the tomatoes into boiling water for 30 seconds, then refresh in cold water. Peel away the skins and chop the flesh roughly. Leave to one side.

Heat 1 tsp coconut oil in a large saucepan and cook the onion, garlic and spices for 5–10 minutes until soft and the onions are translucent.

Remove the pumpkin from the oven. Scoop out the flesh from the wedges and put it in the saucepan. Add the tomato flesh and the remaining ingredients.

Bring to the boil, then reduce the heat and simmer over a low heat for 20–30 minutes until the vegetables are cooked through.

Cool slightly, then purée using a blender or food processor. Return the soup to the pan until ready to serve. Adjust the seasoning to taste, and serve.

Nutritional information per serving: 85 kcals, 2.8g fat, 10g net carbohydrates, 2.1g protein

Carrot and Courgette Soup

I worked for a charity as a nutritionist many years ago and wrote a small recipe book for them. I used to go into people's homes and help them change their diets. This recipe will always remind me of a lady I met. She didn't cook, and this was one of the first recipes she made. She was so impressed with her newly found skill that she made it every day. As delicious as this soup is, I wanted her to expand her repertoire, so I worked very hard to get her to try other things!

■ Double up and freeze

Serves 4
    1 tsp coconut oil or olive oil
    1 red onion, chopped
    1 garlic clove, crushed
    3 carrots, evenly diced

3 courgettes, evenly diced

1 sweet potato, evenly diced

3cm piece of fresh ginger, peeled and grated

600ml vegetable stock

3 tsp thyme leaves or 1 tsp dried thyme

1 tsp paprika

buckwheat, spelt or low-carb, grain-free bread, to serve

Heat the oil in a saucepan over a medium heat and cook the onion and garlic for 1 minute. Add the carrots, courgettes and sweet potato, and cook for a further 2 minutes to soften. Add the ginger and cook for 1 minute.

Add the remaining ingredients and bring to the boil, then reduce the heat and simmer for 20–30 minutes until the vegetables are soft.

This soup is lovely as a chunky soup, but if you want to have a smooth soup, cool it slightly then purée using a blender or food processor. Return the soup to the pan and reheat. Serve with bread.

Nutritional information per serving: 141 kcals, 4g fat, 21g net carbohydrates, 2.8g protein

Roasted Creamy Tomato Soup

I first made this as a non-vegan version with mascarpone instead of coconut cream. Both options work well, but what makes this soup so lovely is the roasting of the tomatoes and onions. I do a lot of work with schools and I decided to get ten 7–10-year-olds to make a five- course meal from scratch, serving it to the local mayor and governors. It was a huge success, with the mayor declaring this was the best soup he had ever tasted.

■ Double up and freeze

Serves 6

  600g tomatoes, quartered

  2 garlic cloves, peeled and left whole

  1 large red onion, quartered

  1 red pepper, deseeded and quartered

  1 carrot, cut into batons

  3 thyme sprigs

  3 tbsp coconut oil, melted, or olive oil

  2 tbsp balsamic vinegar

  seasoning

  400ml vegetable stock

  10 sun-dried tomatoes, without oil

  3 tbsp sun-dried tomato paste

  3 tbsp coconut cream

Preheat the oven to 170°C (150°C fan oven) Gas 3. Put the tomatoes, garlic and vegetables in a roasting tin, then put the thyme sprigs in between them.

Mix the coconut oil with the vinegar and sprinkle it over the vegetables. Season well with salt and pepper, then roast for 30 minutes.

Put the vegetable mixture, including the juice in the roasting tin, into a large saucepan. Add the stock, the sun-dried tomatoes and the sun-dried tomato paste. Purée using a blender or food processor. Return the soup to the pan and add the coconut cream. Bring to the boil, reduce the heat and then bring up to a simmer before serving.

Nutritional information per serving: 184 kcals, 12g fat, 13g net carbohydrates, 2.3g protein

Watercress Soup

We tend to eat only a little watercress in salads, as it can be quite strong, but we really should eat more, because it is full of nutrients. I made the mistake years ago of adding quite a bit to a juice – wow! Never again, as it was so bitter! Thankfully, this recipe is anything but. It is a lovely creamy soup – one of my favourites.

▪ Double up and freeze

Serves 4

1 tsp coconut oil or olive oil
1 red onion, diced
1 garlic clove, roughly chopped
1 celery stick, diced
1 large potato, diced
600ml vegetable stock
250g watercress, chopped
3 tbsp coconut cream
a pinch of finely grated nutmeg
a squeeze of lemon juice, to taste
ground black pepper

Heat the oil in a saucepan over a medium heat and cook the onion and garlic for 2 minutes.

Add the celery and potato, and stir to combine, then cook for 2 minutes.

Add the vegetable stock and bring to the boil, then reduce the heat and simmer for 10 minutes or until the potato is cooked.

Add the watercress and stir to ensure that it is submerged, then cook for 5 minutes.

Cool the soup slightly, then purée using a blender or food processor.

Return the soup to the pan. Add the coconut cream, nutmeg and lemon juice. Combine well and season with pepper to taste. Reheat gently when ready to serve.

Nutritional information per serving: 193 kcals, 7.2g fat, 24g net carbohydrates, 5.2g protein

Sweet Potato, Carrot and Parsnip Soup

I don't know about you, but I always seem to have an abundance of root vegetables in my vegetable drawer. This recipe is perfect for using these up, providing a wonderful creamy, warming and nutritious soup, perfect for the winter months.

■ Double up and freeze

Serves 4
   2 tsp coconut oil or olive oil
   1 leek, sliced
   1 garlic clove, crushed
   2 celery sticks, chopped
   2 sweet potatoes, quartered
   3 carrots, roughly chopped
   1 parsnip, roughly chopped
   600ml vegetable stock, plus extra if needed
   1 tsp dried mixed herbs
   1 tsp onion granules
   1 tsp paprika
   ground black pepper
   2 tbsp coconut cream
   chopped parsley or chilli oil, to garnish

Heat the oil in a large saucepan over a medium heat and cook the leeks for 5 minutes or until they start to soften slightly.

Put the garlic and all vegetables into the pan and cook for another 5 minutes, stirring occasionally.

Add the vegetable stock, herbs, onion granules and paprika, then season with pepper. Bring to the boil, then reduce the heat and simmer for 25 minutes or until the vegetables are tender. Add more stock if needed.

Purée using a blender or food processor, then return the soup to the pan and stir in the coconut cream, then reheat. Serve garnished with parsley or a swirl of chilli oil.

Nutritional information per serving: 177 kcals, 5.8g fat, 26g net carbohydrates, 2.8g protein

Leek and Potato Soup

Who doesn't love a creamy leek and potato soup? Most shop-bought versions contain dairy, however, so this is my vegan version of a great family favourite. I like to liquidise the soup before adding some coconut cream to make it extra creamy, but you can make this as a chunky soup. If you do this, make sure that all the vegetables are cut to equal bite-sized pieces to allow an even cook.

■ Double up and freeze

Serves 4
    2 tsp coconut oil or olive oil
    3 leeks, sliced
    2 garlic cloves, crushed
    2 potatoes, cubed

1 celery stick, chopped

750ml vegetable stock

1 tsp onion granules

3 tsp thyme leaves or 1 tsp dried thyme

¼ tsp finely grated nutmeg

3 tbsp coconut cream

seasoning to taste

buckwheat, spelt or low-carb grain-free bread, to serve

Heat the oil in a saucepan over a medium heat and cook the leeks for a few minutes to allow them to soften.

Add the garlic, potatoes and celery and cook for 5 minutes. Add the vegetable stock, onion granules, thyme and nutmeg, and season with salt and pepper.

Bring to the boil, then reduce the heat and simmer for 20 minutes or until the potatoes are soft.

Purée using a blender or food processor, then return the soup to the pan, stir in the coconut cream, season and reheat. Serve with bread.

Nutritional information per serving 210 kcals, 9g fat, 25g net carbohydrates, 4.3g protein

Salads and Dips

Salads are a vital part of a plant-based diet. They enable us to consume more vegetables and add more variety and colour to our plate.

The salads in this chapter are perfect for workday lunches as well as an accompaniment for your evening meals. I encourage you to mix and match the salads. I make up a batch of three different salads and keep these in airtight containers in my fridge for two to three days; for example, Puy Lentil Salad, Potato Salad and the Rainbow Salad can all be made into one meal – delicious with a dollop of hummus. Add a little of each salad to create a very nutritious and colourful lunch.

The dips can be used as an accompaniment or even a meal or snack on their own.

This chapter also includes salsas and dressings, but if you are taking your salad to work, avoid adding the dressing until you are just about to eat the salad, or you may end up with a soggy mess by lunchtime.

Salads

Long gone is the idea that a salad is just a bit of lettuce, tomato and cucumber on the side of a plate. These salads can be a meal on their own, or as a side. When adding green leaves to your salad, avoid the temptation to opt for a single form of lettuce leaf. Try to incorporate a variety of leaves, as they all bring their own nutrient content. Don't be afraid to add your own variations to these recipes. Also, remember that you can eat a lot of vegetables raw. Broccoli, for example, is a wonderful vegetable, packed with nutrients, and it is delicious when the florets are chopped and added to a salad.

Colourful Sprouting Salad

You can make your own sprouted seeds, but I am not the best at trying to grow things, so I buy mine from the local health-food shop. They add a lovely nuttiness to salads and are nutrient dense. I have combined these with a variety of colourful vegetables and salad leaves. I use this salad as a base, adding sliced avocado and my Tofu Burger (page 205), Thai Bean Cakes (page 107) or my Spicy Sweet Potato Balls (page 108) for a tasty nutritious lunch.

Serves 2
    100g sprouted bean and seed mix
    60g mixed salad leaves
    4 spring onions, diced
    ¼ cucumber, diced
    1 small carrot, grated or spiralised
    40g walnuts, roughly crushed

For the dressing:
  2 tbsp avocado oil
  juice of 1 lemon
  seasoning

Put the sprouted bean and seed mix in a bowl and mix with the salad leaves. Add the spring onions, cucumber and carrots, then combine again. Top with the crushed walnuts.

When ready to serve, mix the avocado oil and lemon juice together. Season to taste with salt and pepper and toss with the salad.

Nutritional information per serving: 332 kcals, 29.6g fat, 6.6g net carbohydrates, 7.8g protein

Minted Puy Lentil Salad

I often prepare this salad to add to a basic green salad. It has a nutty flavour and tastes refreshing with the mint. You can make this in advance and it will keep in the fridge for up to two days, making it a perfect addition to your working lunches. It also makes a complementary side dish for a curry. Puy lentils are a good source of fibre and iron.

Serves 4
  300g Puy lentils
  1 tsp coconut oil or olive oil
  1 red onion, finely chopped
  zest and juice of ½ lemon
  2 tbsp finely chopped mint leaves or 2 tsp dried mint,
    or to taste
  seasoning to taste

Cook the Puy lentils in a saucepan of boiling water for 15 minutes or until tender.

Meanwhile, heat the oil in a saucepan over a medium heat and cook the onion for 5 minutes or until it becomes translucent. Remove the pan from the heat and leave to one side.

Drain the lentils in a colander and tip into the saucepan with the onion. Stir in the lemon zest and juice and the mint, then season to taste. Serve hot or cold.

Nutritional information per serving: 154 kcals, 3.4g fat, 19g net carbohydrates, 8.9g protein

Rainbow Rice Salad

This recipe uses brown rice, but you could also add some wild rice or simply swap for cooked quinoa.

Serves 2

80g brown basmati rice, or 250g cooked rice or quinoa
4 spring onions, finely chopped
1 celery stick, finely chopped
1 green pepper, deseeded and diced
50g sugar snap peas, diced
50g mangetouts, diced
50g frozen peas, defrosted
50g tinned sweetcorn, drained and rinsed
1 green apple, cored and diced
seasoning to taste
1 handful of mint leaves, finely chopped
1 handful of parsley leaves, finely chopped
2 tsp nigella seeds

zest and juice of ½ lemon

2–3 tbsp extra virgin olive oil or flax oil, to taste

Rinse the raw rice several times to remove the starch. Drain, then cook the rice in a large saucepan of boiling water for 10 minutes or until tender. Drain in a colander and spread the rice out on a plate to cool quickly.

Put the cooled rice in a bowl and add the vegetables and apple. Combine well.

Season to taste, then add the herbs, nigella seeds and lemon zest and juice, and combine well. Store in the fridge until ready to serve. Just before to serving, stir in the oil. This can be made in advance and stored in the fridge in an airtight container, without any dressing, for up to 3 days.

Nutritional information per serving: 204 kcals, 7.6g fat, 27g net carbohydrates, 4.6g protein

Roasted Vegetable Salad

Serve this as a light meal or double up the recipe and make extra for lunch the next day.

Serves 4

    1–2 garlic cloves, to taste, roughly chopped

    2 red onions, quartered

    1 aubergine, diced

    1 sweet potato, unpeeled, diced

    1 courgette, diced

    1 carrot, diced

    1 red pepper, deseeded and thickly diced

1 yellow pepper, deseeded and thickly diced

3 thyme sprigs

2 tbsp coconut oil, melted, or olive oil

2 tbsp balsamic vinegar

seasoning to taste

75g baby leaf spinach

30g watercress

2 tbsp pumpkin seeds

1 tbsp sunflower seeds

Preheat the oven to 170°C (150°C fan oven) Gas 3. Put garlic, the vegetables, except the spinach and watercress, and the peppers in a roasting tin and add the thyme sprigs.

Drizzle with oil and balsamic vinegar, then season to taste. Roast for 20 minutes.

Put the spinach and watercress in a large bowl. Fold in the roasted vegetables.

Sprinkle with the seeds and serve hot or cold. This will store well in the fridge in an airtight container for up to 3 days.

Nutritional information per serving: 256 kcals, 11g fat, 27g net carbohydrates, 7g protein

Loaded Potato Salad

My mum always packed up a lunch whenever we went on family day trips. Potato salad was always one of my favourites. This recipe is full of extras to add to the flavour as well as increasing the nutrient content. It uses new potatoes, but you can also use sweet potato (but be careful not overcook the sweet potato or you might have a soggy salad). I often eat this combined with two other salads. It adds variety, and the healthy fats from the avocado combined with the complex carbohydrates from the potato keep you feeling fuller for longer.

Serves 4

    800g new potatoes, halved
    1 bunch of spring onions, chopped
    1 celery stick, finely chopped
    1 green pepper, deseeded and finely chopped
    a small handful of chives, chopped
    a small handful of parsley leaves, chopped
    a small handful of mint leaves, chopped

For the dressing:

    2 ripe avocados, flesh scooped from the skin and
        roughly chopped
    4 tbsp vegan mayonnaise
    1 tbsp extra virgin olive oil or avocado oil
    juice of ½ lemon
    seasoning to taste

Ensure the potatoes are all a similar size for even cooking. Put the potatoes in a steamer and steam over a high heat for 15–20 minutes until tender. Leave to cool.

To make the dressing, mash the avocado in a bowl and stir in the mayonnaise, oil and lemon juice. Season to taste.

Put the cold potatoes into a bowl. Add the vegetables and herbs, then combine thoroughly. Toss in the dressing. Store in an airtight container in the fridge for up to 24 hours until ready to eat.

Nutritional information per serving: 410 kcals, 26g fat, 34g net carbohydrates, 6g protein

Traffic-Light Salad with Citrus Dressing

As the name suggests, this is a vibrant, colourful salad. I have added spiralised beetroot, but this is optional.

Serves 4

    300g mixed salad leaves
    1 large carrot, finely grated or spiralised
    1 small raw beetroot (optional), grated or spiralised
    ½ cucumber, diced
    1 small red onion, diced
    150g cherry tomatoes
    a small handful of fresh basil leaves, chopped
    a few dill sprigs, chopped
    a small handful of parsley leaves, chopped
    juice of 1 orange
    juice of 1 lime
    2 tbsp extra virgin olive oil or avocado oil
    seasoning to taste

Put the salad leaves in a serving bowl. Add the carrot, beetroot, cucumber, onion and tomatoes. Add the chopped herbs and combine well.

Put the orange and lime juice in a small bowl and add the oil. Season, then pour the dressing over the salad and toss to combine just before to serving.

Nutritional information per serving: 125 kcals, 7.3g fat, 9.3g net carbohydrates, 2.9g protein

Salad essentials and dips

Add a different dimension to your salads with these salad extras, or they can be used to help fill your favourite sandwiches. I mix and match my meals, keeping a selection of the slaws and dips in my fridge to add colour, flavour and additional texture to my lunch.

Carrot, Walnut and Ginger Slaw

This simple salad can be made even easier by using a food processor to grate the carrot. It's ideal for barbecues or picnics, or to add some colour to a selection of other salads.

Serves 4

4 carrots, grated or spiralised
3 spring onions, finely sliced
50g walnuts, chopped
3cm piece of fresh ginger, peeled and grated
juice of ½ lemon
2 tbsp olive oil
½ tsp soy sauce or coconut aminos
seasoning to taste

Put the carrots and spring onions in a bowl. Add the walnuts and ginger, and stir well.

Make the dressing by combining the lemon juice, oil and soy sauce together. Season, then pour over the carrots. Stir thoroughly.

Store in the fridge for up to 2 days.

Nutritional information per serving: 182 kcals, 15g fat, 6.3g net carbohydrates, 3g protein

Green Chunky Slaw

An alternative to the standard coleslaw, this mixture of crisp green vegetables is absolutely bursting with nutrients. It looks amazing on your plate as an accompaniment to any meal or to serve alongside a green salad and some scarlet tomatoes.

Serves 6

75g white cabbage, finely sliced

50g sugar snap peas, diced

1 celery stick, finely sliced

75g frozen peas, defrosted

50g baby leaf spinach

1 red onion, sliced

a large handful of mint leaves, chopped

zest and juice of 1 lemon

4 tbsp vegan mayonnaise

9 walnuts, roughly chopped

seasoning to taste

Put all the vegetables in a large bowl and combine well. Put the chopped mint in a small bowl and add the lemon zest and juice, and the mayonnaise. Mix well, then season to taste.

Pour the mayonnaise mixture over the vegetables and combine well. Finish with a sprinkle of the chopped walnuts, then serve.

Nutritional Information per serving 151 kcals, 12g fat, 5.6g net carbohydrates, 3.1g protein

Hummus

Although hummus is readily available in the shops, I urge you to make your own, as it will be nutritionally superior and have an amazing flavour. You can also increase your intake of healthy omega-3 fats by making this with flax oil rather than olive oil. Eat hummus as a great dip, or enjoy it on toast. It contains chickpeas, which are rich in fibre, iron, vitamin B6, magnesium and potassium. If you can leave the hummus to rest, the flavour will improve.

Makes about 300g
    400g can chickpeas, drained and rinsed
    1–3 garlic cloves, to taste, peeled and left whole
    1 tbsp tahini
    2–3 tbsp olive oil or flax oil
    juice of ½ lemon

Put the chickpeas into a blender or food processor and add 1 garlic clove, the tahini, 2 tbsp oil and half the lemon juice. Whizz until smooth. Add more lemon juice or olive oil until you get the desired consistency.

If you taste this and think that it is not garlicky enough, don't be tempted to add more until you have let it rest for at least 20 minutes, then taste it again before adding more.

Store in an airtight container in the fridge for up to 4 days.

Nutritional information per 100g: 159 kcals, 11g fat, 8.8g net carbohydrates, 5.3g protein

Variation: Good flavour combinations include lemon and coriander; chilli; red pepper; or roasted red onions. Simply add your flavour combination and whizz in a blender until smooth.

Artichoke and Butter Bean Hummus

Hummus is a great way to boost your protein levels and it makes a great snack with some vegetable sticks for dipping. This is a tasty variation of traditional hummus containing nutrient-rich artichokes, which are packed with fibre, potassium and vitamin C.

Makes about 350g
  100g artichoke hearts (from a tin or jar), drained
  200g butter beans, drained and rinsed
  1 garlic clove, roughly chopped
  2 tsp ground cumin
  2 tsp finely chopped mint leaves or ½ tsp dried mint
  4 tbsp olive oil
  2 tbsp lemon juice
  1 tbsp tahini
  seasoning to taste

Put all the ingredients into a blender or food processor and whizz until it forms a lovely creamy purée. Season to taste.
  Store in an airtight container in the fridge for up to 4 days.

Nutritional information per 15g serving: 22 kcals, 1.5g fat, 1.1g net carbohydrates, 0.7g protein

Roasted Beetroot Hummus

The colour alone of this hummus will seduce you. Its vibrant pink looks amazing, and it is a match made in heaven when coupled with the green of guacamole (on page 143). You can roast the beetroot in advance. You could also double up the roasted beetroot and use half to make my Roasted Beetroot Falafels on page 159.

Makes about 380g
  2 small raw beetroot, peeled and cut into wedges
  2–3 tbsp olive oil or flax oil
  400g tin chickpeas, drained and rinsed
  1–3 garlic cloves, to taste
  juice of ½ lemon
  1 tbsp tahini

Preheat the oven to 180°C (160°C fan oven) Gas 4. Put the beetroot wedges into a roasting tin and drizzle with 1 tbsp of the oil. Roast for 30 minutes. Remove from the oven and leave to cool.

Put the beetroot into a blender or food processor and add the chickpeas, 1 garlic clove, half the lemon juice and the tahini, and whizz until smooth. Add more lemon juice or olive oil until you get the desired consistency.

If you taste this and think that it is not garlicky enough, don't be tempted to add more until you have let it rest for at least 20 minutes, then taste it again before adding more.

Store in an airtight container in the fridge for up to 4 days.

Nutritional information per 100g: 167 kcals, 11g fat, 10g net carbohydrates, 5.6g protein

Guacamole

Fresh guacamole is far superior in taste and nutritional values to shop-bought kinds and it really only takes minutes to prepare. Guacamole has a base of avocado, with its abundance of healthy fats, and it's a great way to use these exotic fruits up when they become very ripe.

Enjoy guacamole with salads, on toast, in a sandwich or as a side dish for your spicy chilli.

Makes 600g
  3 ripe avocados, flesh scooped from the skin
  juice of ½ lemon or lime, plus extra if needed
  1–2 green chillies, to taste, deseeded and finely chopped
    (see below)
  1 tomato, diced
  3 spring onions, diced
  a small handful of coriander leaves, finely chopped
  1 tbsp extra virgin olive oil
  seasoning to taste

Mash the avocado flesh in a large bowl. Add half the lemon juice and the remaining ingredients, and combine well.

Taste and adjust the seasoning, adding more lemon juice if you wish. Store covered in the fridge and eat soon after preparation.

Nutritional information per 100g: 155 kcals, 15g fat, 2.2g net carbohydrates, 1.5g protein

Chillies – to seed or not to seed?: The seeds of chillies hold much of the heat, so for moderate heat they are best deseeded, but if you like lots of chilli heat, do not deseed them.

Salsa

Serve a salsa as a delicious side dish to add flavour and a kick of chilli heat to any meal. It can add a nice touch to your everyday salads, but it can also be a great served alongside a savoury dish as a relish.

Serves 4

4 tomatoes, chopped

¼ cucumber, diced

1–2 chillies, to taste, deseeded and finely chopped

1 red pepper, deseeded and finely chopped

4 spring onions, finely chopped

a small handful of coriander leaves, finely chopped

1–2 garlic cloves, to taste, crushed

1 tbsp balsamic vinegar

2 tbsp olive oil

zest and juice of ½ lemon, or to taste

seasoning to taste

Put the tomatoes, cucumber and chillies in a bowl and add the pepper, spring onions, coriander and garlic, then mix them together.

Add the balsamic vinegar, olive oil and lemon zest, then mix well and add lemon juice to taste. Season with salt and pepper.

Leave the salsa to settle for at least 15 minutes to allow the flavours to infuse before serving.

Nutritional information per serving: 103 kcals, 6.8g fat, 6.4g net carbohydrates, 1.6g protein

Side Dishes

This chapter provides a selection of dishes to accompany meals. You will find the versatile cauliflower rice here: a simple and great way to boost your meal with added vegetables. I have also included a simple way to cook quinoa, as I have found that many people are unsure about the best way of cooking it.

Cauliflower Rice

This speedy vegetable side dish is popular with vegans and those following low-carb diets. There are two ways I cook this: one uses the microwave and the other is to sauté it. You can also steam cauliflower or put whole florets on a baking tray and roast them before zapping them in a food processor.

Serves 4
  1 whole cauliflower, cut into florets
  1 tsp coconut oil or olive oil (if sauté cooking)
  seasoning to taste

Put the cauliflower into a food processor or electric chopper and pulse for a few seconds until the cauliflower resembles rice. (If you don't have a processor you can grate the cauliflower, but it is messy and more time-consuming.)

Microwave cooking When ready to cook, put the cauliflower in a lidded container, without any water and pop it into your microwave. Cook on full power for 5–8 minutes depending on your microwave. Stir halfway through cooking to ensure an even cook.

Remove and fluff up with a fork, season and serve immediately.

Sauté cooking Heat 1 tbsp coconut oil or olive oil in a saucepan over a medium heat. Add the cauliflower and toss gently for 5–8 minutes until heated through and softened. Season and serve immediately.

Nutritional information per serving: 39 kcals, 0.4g fat, 4.8g net carbo-hydrates, 2.8g protein

---

Tips for cooking cauliflower

- **Make in bulk** Whizz up a few cauliflowers at a time and put the uncooked processed cauliflower rice into freezer bags. You can use this from frozen – just add to the saucepan and cook through.
- **Cauliflower mash** If you want to make mash, simply prepare the cauliflower as you would for cauliflower rice. When hot, mash the cauliflower as much as you can with a fork – it will soon reduce. Traditionally, you would add butter to make it creamy, but you can use plant-based milk or coconut cream for a vegan alternative. Season it with salt and pepper to taste. (You can also make a lovely

mash in the same way using celeriac, parsnip, butternut squash or swede.)

- **Roasted cauliflower** You can roast a whole cauliflower and then blitz it to form cauliflower rice or cauliflower mash, but it is also amazing when thickly sliced to form cauliflower steaks. Preheat the oven to 180°C (160°C fan oven) Gas 4. Put the cauliflower (whole or sliced) onto a baking tray. Add 3 tbsp coconut oil or olive oil. You can also add flavour with a variety of herbs and spices: I like to add thyme leaves and a few crushed garlic cloves. For a spicy touch, add some chilli flakes, a sprinkle of paprika and some ground coriander. Roast the cauliflower steaks for 20 minutes or 30–40 minutes for a whole cauliflower, depending on size. Blitz it to make cauliflower rice or eat it as a roasted vegetable.

Curried Cauliflower Rice

Cauliflower works fantastically well with spices, so here's how to add a little kick to your cauliflower rice.

Serves 4

   1 whole cauliflower, cut into florets
   1 tbsp coconut oil or olive oil
   1 small red onion, finely chopped
   2 garlic cloves, crushed
   1 red chilli, deseeded and finely chopped
   1 tsp ground turmeric
   1 tbsp curry powder
   seasoning to taste

Put the cauliflower into a food processor or electric chopper and pulse for a few minutes until the cauliflower resembles rice. (If you don't have a processor you can grate the cauliflower, but it is messy and more time-consuming.)

Heat the oil in a saucepan over a medium heat and add the onion, garlic, chilli and spices. Combine well, then add the cauliflower.

Cook, stirring, for 5–8 minutes until heated through and softened. Season then serve immediately.

Nutritional information per serving: 82 kcals, 3.8g fat, 6.7g net carbohydrates, 3.4g protein

Perfect Quinoa

Some people worry about cooking quinoa, but it is very simple and it makes the perfect switch for rice or couscous.

Serves 2
  100g quinoa
  seasoning

Put the quinoa in a sieve and rinse well under cold running water. Tip into a saucepan and add 250ml water. Season with a little salt.

Cook over a medium-low heat for 10–15 minutes until the grains have swollen. Check occasionally to ensure it does not boil dry, and add more water if necessary.

Remove from the heat and stir to fluff up the grains. Season with pepper and serve as a side dish or cool and add to a salad.

Nutritional information per serving: 160 kcals, 2.6g fat, 26g net carbohydrates, 7g protein

Variation: Turmeric is a great healthy spice to add to quinoa. It is a wonderful anti-inflammatory due to its active ingredient curcumin – it also has a brilliant colour. Curcumin works best when combined with pepper, so add 1 tsp ground turmeric and a generous sprinkle of black pepper to the quinoa and water before cooking, to make a lovely vibrant yellow quinoa.

Roasted Vegetables

Practically any vegetable can be roasted to make a delicious side dish. I like to add fresh herbs, such as thyme or rosemary, along with garlic and plenty of salt and pepper. You can combine olive oil with balsamic vinegar to create a more caramelised flavour. You can also add chillies and chilli flakes for a hot kick.

Serves 4

   3 garlic cloves, peeled and halved
   2 red onions, cut into wedges
   1 courgette, cut into thick slices
   1 aubergine, cut into thick slices
   1 sweet potato, unpeeled, cut into thick slices
   1 red pepper, deseeded and cut into wedges or
      thick slices
   3 tomatoes, cut into wedges
   4 thyme sprigs
   seasoning
   2 tbsp olive oil

Preheat the oven to 180°C (160°C fan oven) Gas 4. Put the garlic, vegetables, pepper and tomatoes into a roasting tin. Add the thyme and season well with salt and pepper.

Drizzle over the oil and combine well, ensuring the vegetables are evenly coated, and then spread them out evenly in the tin.

Roast for 20–25 minutes until golden and tender. Serve immediately.

Nutritional information per serving: 198 kcals, 7.3g fat, 25g net carbohydrates, 3.9g protein

Celeriac Chips

These celery-flavoured chips have a lovely taste that is very different from white potatoes, and they are also less carb-heavy. You can fry these chips, but as I like to avoid processed oils, especially vegetable and seed oils, it is far better to bake them in the oven. (You can use the same recipe with sweet potato, which is lovely when combined with the chilli flakes.)

Serves 2

    1 large celeriac
    1 tsp paprika
    2 tbsp vegan Parmesan (see page 237)
    ground black pepper
    ½ tsp of chilli flakes (optional)
    2–3 tbsp coconut oil, melted, or olive oil

To prepare the celeriac, cut off the top and bottom, then turn onto a flat edge and run the knife down the sides to remove the hard outer edge. Cut into thick fingers.

Put the celeriac in a saucepan, cover with the boiling water and boil for 8–10 minutes until tender when tested with a knife. Drain in a colander and tip into a bowl.

Sprinkle with the paprika, my homemade vegan Parmesan and black pepper. If you like a chilli kick, add the chilli flakes.

Drizzle with the oil and combine well. Tip onto a baking sheet, and check that none of the celeriac fingers are overlapping. Bake for 30 minutes or until golden, then serve.

Nutritional information per serving: 225 kcals, 18g fat, 4.4g net carbohydrates, 6.4g protein

Spicy Rice

Don't be put off by the number of ingredients in this recipe, as this is a really nice, simple recipe that can be used as a side dish, a salad or a main meal. I like to combine brown rice with wild rice because it gives it a lovely nutty flavour and texture. Serve hot or cold.

Serves 4

1 tsp coconut oil or olive oil

1 red onion, diced

2 garlic cloves, crushed

4cm piece of fresh ginger, peeled and grated

1 red pepper, deseeded and diced

1 red chilli, deseeded and finely chopped

1 tsp ground coriander

1 tsp ground cardamom

1 tsp ground cumin

1 tsp ground turmeric

½ tsp finely grated nutmeg

250g brown basmati rice

50g wild rice

550ml water or vegetable stock

1 cinnamon stick

1 bay leaf

75g peas, defrosted if frozen

50g sweetcorn, defrosted if frozen, or tinned, drained
   and rinsed

25g flaked almonds

a small handful of coriander leaves

Heat the oil in a large saucepan or flameproof casserole over a medium
heat and cook the onion, garlic, ginger, pepper and chilli for 2 minutes
to soften.

Add the ground spices and the nutmeg, and cook for 2 minutes.

Add the rice and wild rice, then stir well to ensure the flavours blend
through. Add the water, the cinnamon stick and bay leaf. Cover with a
lid and cook over a medium heat for 15 minutes.

Turn off the heat. Add the peas, sweetcorn, flaked almonds and
coriander leaves. Stir and cover again. Leave for 10 minutes. Loosen
with a fork before serving.

Nutritional information per serving: 388 kcals, 8.6g fat, 62g net carbohydrates, 12g protein

Wilted Kale with Garlic and Lemon

Here is a tasty way to serve kale – a super-healthy vegetable, containing
antioxidants. It also contains two carotenoids – lutein and zeaxanthin –
which are beneficial for eye health. You can swap the kale with cavolo
nero (also known as black kale) or even savoy cabbage.

Serves 4

    1 tbsp coconut oil or olive oil

    2–3 garlic cloves, to taste, crushed

    zest and juice of 1 lemon, or to taste

    150ml vegetable stock or water

    350g kale, shredded

    seasoning to taste

Heat the oil in a saucepan over a medium heat and cook the garlic and lemon zest for 1 minute.

Add the stock and the kale. Bring to the boil then cover and reduce the heat. Simmer for 5–8 minutes until the kale is cooked and reduced.

Season with salt, pepper and lemon juice to taste. Stir well until combined. Serve immediately.

Nutritional Information per serving 83 kcals, 6.6g fat, 1.8g Net Carbohydrates, 3.3g protein

Comforting Hot Green Salad

This is my fall-back green salad when I don't fancy a cold salad and prefer something warm but extra-tasty. Use your steamer to preserve all the nutrients.

Serves 4

    150g asparagus

    150g green beans, cut into short lengths

    150g peas

    150g Tenderstem broccoli

    1 tbsp coconut oil or olive oil

    75g walnuts

For the dressing:

    4 tbsp extra virgin olive oil

    2 tbsp white wine vinegar

    2 tsp finely chopped mint leaves or ½ tsp dried mint

    ground black pepper

Snap off the coarse ends of the asparagus and discard them. Cut the spears into short lengths. Put the asparagus and remaining vegetables in a steamer and steam over a high heat for 5 minutes until tender. (Alternatively, if you don't have a steamer you can blanch them in a saucepan of boiling water for no more than 4 minutes.) You want the vegetables to be slightly crunchy, not soft and soggy.

While the vegetables are cooking, make the dressing by combining all the ingredients, adjusting the proportions to suit your own personal taste.

Heat the oil in a small saucepan over a medium heat and add the walnuts. Toss gently in the hot oil until they darken slightly. Remove and leave to one side until the vegetables are cooked.

Put the steamed vegetables in a bowl, add the walnuts and pour over the dressing. Combine well before serving.

Nutritional information per serving: 316 kcals, 26g fat, 7.4g net carbohydrates, 8.6g protein

Weekend Lunches

Weekends are a time to enjoy spending a little more time in the kitchen to create a meal that's a bit different from your midweek favourites. You might also find some of these work well in combination to create a lovely evening meal – my favourite is Spicy Puy Lentil and Quinoa Tabbouleh with Roasted Beetroot Falafels, drizzled with tahini (page 67).

Some of the recipes in this chapter can be made in advance. You will see them marked as 'Get ahead'. These are perfect if you want to plan ahead and make dishes in advance.

Green Bean and Cashew Stir-fry

This makes a perfect light lunch, or you can use this as a side dish for a main meal. You can use asparagus instead of green beans when it's in season.

Serves 2

2 tbsp dry sherry

1 tbsp soy sauce or coconut aminos

1 tbsp red wine vinegar

2 tsp coconut oil or olive oil

8 spring onions, chopped

1 celery stick, chopped

2 garlic cloves, crushed

3cm piece of fresh ginger, peeled and grated

1–2 green chillies, deseeded and chopped

150g green beans

150g mangetouts

75g cashew nuts

a small handful of coriander leaves, roughly chopped

Put the sherry in a small bowl and add the soy sauce and vinegar. Mix together, then leave to stand.

Heat the oil in a wok or large saucepan over a medium heat. Add the spring onions, celery, garlic, ginger and chillies, and cook for 2 minutes.

Add the beans, mangetouts and cashew nuts, and cook for 3 minutes.

Pour over the sherry mixture and toss the ingredients for 1 minute until coated. Add the coriander and serve immediately.

Nutritional information per serving: 336 kcals, 21g fat, 15g net carbohydrates, 14g protein

Spicy Puy Lentil and Quinoa Tabbouleh

Made with protein-rich quinoa and lentils, this is perfect for a summer's day barbecue as a side dish or for a light lunch. The flavour is enhanced by the combination of the sweetness of the tomatoes and a light hit of chilli.

■ Get ahead – this dish can be prepared in advance

Serves 4

   150g Puy lentils
   200g quinoa, rinsed (see page 149)
   1 tsp ground turmeric
   1–2 red chillies, to taste, deseeded and finely chopped
   1 small red onion, finely chopped
   200g cherry tomatoes, halved
   a handful of mint leaves, finely chopped
   a small handful of coriander leaves, finely chopped

For the dressing:

   3 tbsp extra virgin olive oil
   juice of 1 lemon
   2 tsp finely chopped mint leaves or ½ tsp dried mint
   seasoning to taste

Put the lentils in a saucepan and cover with boiling water. Add a touch of salt if you like them seasoned.

Put the quinoa in a saucepan and add 350ml water. Add the turmeric. Bring both saucepans to the boil, then reduce the heat and simmer for 12–15 minutes until tender.

Drain both saucepans in a colander and tip the lentils and quinoa into a large serving bowl. Leave to cool. Add the remaining ingredients.

Put all the dressing ingredients in a small bowl and mix together well. When ready to serve, pour the dressing over the lentil mixture and combine well.

Nutritional information per serving: 336 kcals, 13g fat, 38g net carbohydrates, 12g protein

Roasted Beetroot Falafels

The bright colour of these falafels is stunning – it just screams healthy! They are a perfect alfresco food – so easy to make and delicious served with a selection of salad leaves. This dish is high in manganese, which offers a range of benefits including bone and joint health, cognitive function, and sugar and hormone balancing.

- Get ahead – this dish can be prepared in advance
- Double up and freeze

Serves 4

    2 raw beetroot, peeled and cut into wedges
    1 tbsp coconut oil, melted, or olive oil
    1 tbsp balsamic vinegar
    2 × 400g tins chickpeas, drained and rinsed
    3–4 garlic cloves, to taste, crushed
    1 small red onion, peeled
    2 tbsp tahini, plus extra to serve
    2 tsp ground cumin
    1 tsp ground coriander
    ½–1 tsp chilli powder, to taste
    a squeeze of lemon juice
    seasoning to taste
    green leaf salad, to serve

Preheat the oven to 180°C (160°C fan oven) Gas 4. Put the beetroot in a roasting tin and drizzle over the oil and balsamic vinegar. Season with salt and pepper. Roast for 30–40 minutes until tender.

Put the beetroot into a food processor and add the remaining falafel ingredients, then whizz to a moist paste.

Form into golf-ball sized balls or flat patties and put onto a baking tray. Cook in the oven for 20 minutes. Serve on a bed of green leaf salad and drizzle with some tahini.

Nutritional information per serving: 237 kcals, 9g fat, 23g net carbohydrates, 12g protein

Creamy Masoor Dahl

This is so easy to make and costs very little. This version is mild and creamy, but you can make it more spicy by adding a few chopped chillies.

■ Get ahead – this dish can be prepared in advance
■ Double up and freeze

Serves 4
  2 tsp coconut oil or olive oil
  1 onion, finely chopped
  2 garlic cloves, crushed
  3cm piece of fresh ginger, peeled and finely chopped
  1 red pepper, deseeded and finely chopped
  1 tbsp mild curry powder, or to taste
  1 tsp ground turmeric
  2 tomatoes, finely chopped
  100g red lentils
  1 tbsp tomato purée
  3 tbsp coconut cream
  seasoning to taste
  2 tsp desiccated coconut

Heat the oil in a saucepan over a medium heat and cook the onion, garlic, ginger and pepper for 5–8 minutes until it starts to soften.

Add the curry powder, turmeric and tomatoes, and cook for 2 minutes. (You can adjust the curry powder to suit your personal taste; this recipe is quite mild.)

Add the lentils and tomato purée, and cover with 400ml water. Bring to the boil then reduce the heat and simmer gently for 10 minutes or until the lentils start to soften and open up. Add more water if necessary.

Stir in the coconut cream and season with salt and pepper to taste. Sprinkle with desiccated coconut and serve.

Nutritional information per serving: 202 kcals, 6.9g fat, 23g net carbohydrates, 8.5g protein

Variations: You can also turn this dish into a nourishing soup by adding more liquid until you get the fluidity you desire. You can also follow the same recipe and switch the red lentils for yellow split peas, although you may need to add more liquid as they cook.

Garlic Butter Bean Mash-Up

The creaminess of butter beans paired with garlic is a match made in heaven. You can use spinach or kale if you don't have any cavolo nero, but do try to find it if you can, because it has a richer taste than standard kale.

Serves 4
    2 tsp coconut oil or olive oil
    6 spring onions, chopped
    3 garlic cloves, crushed
    60g flaked almonds
    2 × 400g tins butter beans, drained and rinsed

100g cavolo nero, shredded
black pepper to taste
1–2 tbsp extra virgin olive oil, to taste
3 tbsp vegan Parmesan (see page 237)

Heat the oil in a saucepan over a medium heat and add the spring onions, garlic and flaked almonds. Cook for 2 minutes, then add the butter beans.

Add the cavolo nero, a little at a time, and stir between each addition. Reduce the heat to low and cook for 8–10 minutes to help soften the kale. Season with black pepper.

When ready to serve, drizzle with the olive oil then sprinkle over some homemade vegan Parmesan.

Nutritional information per serving: 418 kcals, 20g fat, 30g net carbohydrates, 22g protein

Broccoli and Leek Tart

This is perfect for a weekend lunch, either hot or cold, or even a packed lunch, and it is well worth doubling the recipe to plan ahead. I make it in a 23cm tart tin, but it works really well in individual tart tins, which are ideal for a packed lunch. The recipe uses soaked cashew nuts to form the creamy base – these need to be soaked for at least 1 hour.

■ Get ahead – this dish can be prepared in advance
■ Double up and freeze

Serves 8
120g cashew nuts
250g buckwheat or spelt flour, plus extra for dusting

125g coconut oil, chilled and cut into small pieces, plus extra
    for greasing and frying
200g Tenderstem broccoli
2 leeks, finely chopped
black pepper
4 tbsp arrowroot
3 tbsp nutritional yeast flakes
green salad, to serve

Put the cashew nuts in a bowl and cover with water. Leave for at least 1 hour.

Put the flour in a food processor and add the coconut oil. Whizz until the mix resembles breadcrumbs. (Alternatively, rub the coconut oil gently into the flour using your fingers, but try not to handle the mixture too much.)

Add 3–5 tablespoons cold water, a little at a time (you may not need it all) and mix with a fork until it comes together. Use your hands to form a dough. Wrap the dough in cling film and put it in the fridge to rest until needed.

Preheat the oven to 200°C (180°C fan oven) Gas 6 and grease a 23cm flan tin. Roll out the pastry on a lightly floured work surface to a bit larger than the tin, and line the tin. Put a sheet of baking parchment over the pastry and cover with baking beans. Bake in the oven for 10 minutes. Remove the baking beans and parchment, and cook for a further 10 minutes until it starts to colour. Remove the pastry case from the oven and turn the oven down to 180°C (160°C fan oven) Gas 4.

While the pastry is baking, put the Tenderstem in a steamer and steam over a high heat for 10 minutes or until starting to soften slightly.

Heat the coconut oil in a saucepan over a medium heat and cook the leeks until they start to soften. Add the Tenderstem, season well with black pepper and put to one side.

Drain the cashew nuts in a colander and put them in a blender or food processor with 150ml water. Add the arrowroot and nutritional yeast flakes, and season with black pepper. Whizz to form a creamy sauce.

Put the leeks and Tenderstem into the tartlet, then pour over the creamy sauce. Cook in the oven for 20–25 minutes until golden. Serve hot or cold with a green salad.

Nutritional information per serving 406 kcals, 24g fat, 33g net carbohydrates, 11g protein

Variation: You can also make this recipe in individual tartlet tins, in which case they will take 15–20 minutes to cook.

Tuscan-Style Beans

Although simple to make, this is full of flavour and makes a sustaining lunch. It can be made in advance and stores well in the fridge.

▪ Get ahead – this dish can be prepared in advance
▪ Double up and freeze

Serves 6

1 tsp coconut oil or olive oil
1 large red onion, chopped
2–3 garlic cloves, to taste, roughly chopped
1 red pepper, deseeded and diced
1 celery stick, diced
2 × 400g tins chopped tomatoes
2 × 400g tins borlotti or cannellini beans (or one of each), drained and rinsed
2 tsp thyme leaves or ½ tsp dried thyme

1 tsp dried marjoram

1 tbsp chopped parsley leaves or 1 tsp dried parsley

seasoning to taste

chopped parsley leaves, to garnish

Heat the oil in a saucepan over a medium heat and cook the onion, garlic, pepper and celery for 5 minutes to soften. Add the remaining ingredients and combine well.

Bring to the boil, then reduce the heat and simmer for 10 minutes.

Season well with salt and pepper to taste. Serve garnished with a sprinkle of fresh parsley. Store in the fridge for up to 3 days.

Nutritional information per serving: 160 kcals, 1.3g fat, 21g net carbohydrates, 9.6g protein

Evening Meals for Crazy Days

These are the days when you are hungry and frazzled, and the last thing you feel like doing is cooking a meal, but before you ditch everything and run for the nearest takeaway, read on.

It's best to be prepared for evening meals when you won't have much time to cook, so several of these recipes involve some planning ahead to make it all run smoothly. That is the key to good nutrition and easy meals. I encourage you, if you have a freezer, to double up some of the recipes and freeze them. Think of this as a way of creating your own ready-meals for when those days are really, really busy! A slow cooker comes in handy for prepping some dishes in the morning and leaving them to cook for the day, and some recipes can prepped the night before.

Thai Green Curry

Using Thai flavourings opens up a new dimension in cooking. This fragrant curry is milder than an Indian curry and therefore more appealing to those who don't like too much spicy heat. Some supermarkets sell complete packs of the fresh Thai herbs, but if you can't find them, opt for a good-quality Thai green curry paste. I serve this with brown basmati rice, cauliflower rice or, for added protein, quinoa.

Serves 4
    1 head of broccoli, cut into florets
    1 tbsp coconut oil or olive oil
    1 bunch of spring onions, diced
    1 red pepper, deseeded and diced
    400g tofu, diced
    3 tbsp coconut cream
    80g green beans, cut in half
    75g pak choi, roughly chopped
    75g baby leaf spinach
    brown rice, quinoa or cauliflower rice (page 146), to serve

For the Thai green curry paste:
    2 garlic cloves, roughly chopped
    2 green chillies, or to taste, deseeded
    1 small red onion, roughly chopped
    3cm piece of fresh ginger, peeled and grated
    2 lemongrass stalks, tough outer covering removed
    4 kaffir lime leaves
    2 tbsp almond butter
    a small handful of coriander leaves
    2 tbsp coconut oil or olive oil, plus extra if needed

Put the broccoli in a steamer and steam over a high heat for 10 minutes until just tender but still with some bite. Meanwhile, put all the Thai paste ingredients into a blender or food processor and whizz until it forms a very smooth paste. Add more oil if you need more liquid. Leave to one side.

Meanwhile, heat the 1 tbsp coconut oil in a saucepan over a

medium heat, and cook the spring onions, pepper and tofu for 5–8 minutes or until the tofu is golden.

Add the Thai paste and coconut cream, and combine well.

Add the steamed broccoli florets, the green beans, pak choi and spinach, and cook for 10 minutes. Serve with brown rice.

Nutritional information per serving 350 kcals, 21g fat, 12g net carbohydrates, 24g protein

Garlic Mushroom and Spinach Butternut Spaghetti

For this quick-and-easy meal packed with flavour, butternut squash is made into spaghetti strands using a spiraliser or using a Y-shaped vegetable peeler (see tip below). You can of course opt for a buckwheat, spelt or rice spaghetti or pasta to accompany dishes if you prefer, but I love spiralised butternut squash: after all, it is another vegetable to add to your plate. You could use courgette spaghetti if you fancy a change in flavour.

Serves 4

2 tsp coconut oil or olive oil

3 garlic cloves, crushed

1 small red onion, finely chopped

250g chestnut mushrooms, quartered

1 tbsp chopped chives

a small handful of parsley leaves, chopped

1 tsp dried tarragon

zest and juice of ½ lemon

3 tbsp coconut cream

300g butternut squash, spiralised or cut into slithers using a
    vegetable peeler (see below)

75g baby leaf spinach, roughly chopped
seasoning to taste

Heat the oil in a large saucepan over a medium heat and cook the garlic, onion and mushrooms for 5–8 minutes until they start to soften.

Add the herbs, lemon zest and juice, and coconut cream, and cook for 3 minutes. Add the butternut and spinach, and cook until soft and the spinach starts to wilt. Season well with salt and pepper to taste, and serve immediately.

Nutritional information per serving: 114 kcals, 6.4g fat, 7.6g net carbohydrates, 4.6g protein

Making spaghetti from vegetables: Vegetable spaghetti looks bright and tastes wonderfully fresh served with all kinds of dishes. If you want to make this regularly, you could buy a spiraliser. Otherwise, use a Y-shaped vegetable peeler to shave off strips, which can be left as they are or cut into finer strands if you wish. Alternatively, you can cut the vegetable into thin slices and then into matchstick strips, although this will take longer.

Simple Vegan Chilli

Despite the long list of ingredients, this really is a simple recipe. Just throw it all into your saucepan and wait for the magic to happen. You can serve it with some brown basmati rice or, if you prefer to keep your carbohydrates in check, some cauliflower rice (see page 146).

■ Get ahead – this dish can be prepared in advance
■ Double up and freeze

Serves 6

  1 tsp coconut oil or olive oil

  1 red onion, diced

  2 garlic cloves, finely chopped

  1 red pepper, deseeded and diced

  1 aubergine, thickly diced

  2 celery sticks, diced

  1 courgette, diced

  1–2 red chillies, to taste, deseeded and finely sliced

  1 tsp dried marjoram

  2 tsp dried oregano

  2 heaped tsp paprika

  1 tsp ground cumin

  1 tsp ground coriander

  1–2 tsp chilli powder, to taste

  seasoning to taste

  2 tbsp sun-dried tomato paste

  400g tin kidney beans, drained and rinsed

  400g tin cannellini beans, drained and rinsed

  400g tin chopped tomatoes

  200ml vegetable stock or water

Heat the oil in a saucepan over a medium heat and cook the onion, garlic, pepper, aubergine, celery, courgette and chillies for 2 minutes.

Add the herbs and spices, and season. Add the remaining ingredients. Bring to the boil, then reduce the heat and simmer for 15–20 minutes, stirring occasionally. Serve.

Nutritional information per serving: 223 kcals, 8.1g fat, 22g net carbohydrates, 8.6g protein

Broccoli and Tofu Stir-Fry

A stir-fry is so fast to get together. If you have time in the morning, you can marinate the tofu in the soy sauce and leave it in the fridge until you make your evening meal – it gives the tofu a little more potency. Serve the stir-fry on a bed of brown rice, quinoa or cauliflower rice, but remember that a stir-fry is so quick to cook that you will need to start cooking your rice or quinoa first.

Serves 4

    2–3 tsp coconut oil or olive oil
    400g organic tofu, diced
    2 dashes plus 2 tbsp soy sauce or coconut aminos
    6 spring onions, sliced
    2–3 garlic cloves, to taste, chopped
    3cm piece of fresh ginger, peeled and finely chopped
    1–2 green chillies, to taste, deseeded and finely chopped
    300g head of broccoli, cut into florets
    200g green beans or asparagus
    1 red or green pepper, deseeded and sliced
    25g flaked almonds
    seasoning to taste
    brown rice, quinoa or cauliflower rice (page 146), and soy
        sauce (optional), to serve

Heat 2 tsp of the oil in a saucepan over a medium heat and cook the tofu with the 2 dashes of soy sauce for 5–8 minutes or until the tofu changes to light brown. Carefully remove the tofu pieces and put to one side.

Add another 1 tsp coconut oil, if needed, and add the spring onions, garlic, ginger and chillies.

Add the broccoli, green beans, pepper and remaining soy sauce, and cook for 5 minutes, then add the tofu and flaked almonds. Continue to cook for 5 minutes or until the broccoli is tender. Season to taste. Serve with rice, with a drizzle of soy sauce, if you like.

Nutritional information per serving 274 kcals, 14g fat, 9g net carbohydrates, 23g protein

Ratatouille

You can't really have a vegan cookbook without including this firm favourite. It is so simple to make but it's absolutely delicious. You can top it with some grilled tofu or simply serve it with some buckwheat bread and a green salad.

Serves 4

1–2 tsp coconut oil or olive oil
1 red onion, sliced
2–3 garlic cloves, to taste, roughly chopped
1 red pepper, deseeded and cut into large dice
1 courgette, cut into large dice
1 aubergine, cut into large dice
3 tomatoes, roughly chopped
2 tbsp sun-dried tomato paste
½ tsp paprika
2 tsp fresh oregano or 1 tsp dried oregano
1 sprig fresh rosemary or ½ tsp dried rosemary
2 tsp thyme leaves or ½ tsp dried thyme
2 tsp chopped basil leaves ½ tsp dried basil
1 tbsp chopped parsley leaves or 1 tsp dried parsley
seasoning to taste
buckwheat bread and a green salad, to serve

Heat the oil in a large saucepan over a medium heat and cook the onion, garlic and pepper for 2 minutes.

Add the courgette and aubergine and cook for 5 minutes then add the tomatoes, tomato paste, paprika and herbs. Season with salt and pepper, and cook gently for 5–10 minutes until the vegetables soften – don't overcook them, as there is nothing worse than a slimy ratatouille. Serve with bread and a green salad.

Nutritional information per serving: 167 kcals, 11g fat, 10g net carbo-hydrates, 3.1g protein

Variations: You can incorporate some baby leaf spinach for the last 1 minute of cooking if you want to include a leafy green. If you want to increase the protein content of the dish, add a tin of chickpeas or butter beans or some toasted nuts.

Tofu Noodle Salad

You can have this meal ready to serve in just 20 minutes, but you could also prepare all the elements separately in advance and serve it cold for a super-quick meal. Tofu is great because it absorbs all the flavours in the dish.

■ Get ahead – this dish can be prepared in advance

Serves 4
  175g vermicelli noodles
  75g frozen peas
  100g green beans, diced
  150g broccoli florets
  50g sweetcorn frozen, or tinned, drained and rinsed

2 tsp coconut oil or olive oil

2 garlic cloves, crushed

2cm piece of fresh ginger, peeled and finely
chopped

1–2 green chillies, to taste, deseeded and
finely chopped

1 bunch of spring onions, chopped

1 red or yellow pepper, deseeded and diced

400g firm tofu, cut into chunks

For the dressing:

2 tbsp soy sauce or coconut aminos

juice of 1 lemon

2 tbsp almond butter or peanut butter

2 tbsp sweet chilli sauce

ground black pepper

Put the noodles in a bowl and pour over boiling water. Leave to stand for 5 minutes, then drain in a colander and rinse with cold water. Drain again and leave to one side.

Half-fill a large saucepan with boiling water over a medium-high heat. Add the peas, green beans, broccoli and sweetcorn. Cook for 5–8 minutes until the broccoli is tender but still firm to the bite.

Rinse immediately in cold water to maintain the freshness, then leave to one side.

Heat the oil in a saucepan over a medium heat. Add the garlic, ginger, chillies, spring onions, pepper and tofu, and cook for 5–8 minutes or until the tofu has browned.

To make the dressing, put all the ingredients in a bowl and whisk well to ensure that they are evenly combined and the nut butter is smooth and free of lumps. Season to taste with black pepper.

When ready to serve, combine all three elements together, then add the dressing, toss together and serve.

Nutritional information per serving: 331 kcals, 17g fat, 17g net carbohydrates, 23g protein

Pesto-Infused Courgette Spaghetti with Asparagus and Spinach

Vibrant green in colour and richly flavoured, pesto goes so well with
asparagus, spinach and courgette with the contrasting colour and
sweetness of cherry tomatoes. To enhance the flavour of the tomatoes,
ensure that they are served at room temperature and not straight from
the fridge. This recipe uses spiralised courgette, but you can also use
spiralised butternut squash. You can double up the pesto recipe and
store it in the fridge for up to one week.

Serves 4
    200g asparagus
    1 tsp coconut oil or olive oil
    1 red onion, diced
    100g baby leaf spinach
    4 courgettes, spiralised or cut into slithers using a vegetable
        peeler (see tip page 169)
    200g cherry tomatoes, halved

For the pesto:
    100g basil leaves (about 3 handfuls)
    2–3 garlic cloves, to taste
    3 tbsp nutritional yeast flakes
    30g pine nuts
    juice of ½ lemon
    4 tbsp extra virgin olive oil
    seasoning

To make the pesto, put the basil, garlic, nutritional yeast flakes, pine nuts and lemon juice into a blender or food processor and whizz to finely chop. Gradually add the oil and 2–3 tbsp water until you reach the desired consistency for your pesto. This needs to be creamy but not runny. Season with salt and pepper to taste.

Snap off the coarse ends of the asparagus and discard them, then cut the spears into thick slices.

Heat the oil in a saucepan over a medium heat and cook the onion and asparagus for 3–4 minutes until the onion begins to soften.

Add the spinach, a little at a time, to help it break down and shrink into the pan. You can add a little hot water if it is being stubborn, but no more than 3 tbsp.

Once the spinach is added, add the spiralised courgettes. Stir in 3–4 tbsp of your pesto, to taste, and cook until the asparagus and courgette are tender.

Remove from the heat and stir in the cherry tomatoes. Serve immediately. The pesto can be stored in an airtight jar in the fridge for 1 week or it can be frozen.

Nutritional information per serving: 226 kcals, 14g fat, 11g net carbohydrates, 10g protein

Sweet Potato and Spinach Curry

You can have this quick-and-easy creamy curry on the table in about 30 minutes. Adjust the spices to suit your own palate, if you wish.

■ Get ahead – this dish can be prepared in advance
■ Double up and freeze

Serves 4

    2 tsp coconut oil or olive oil

    1 large red onion, diced

    1 red pepper, deseeded and diced

    2–3 garlic cloves, to taste, crushed

    1–3 chillies, to taste, deseeded, diced

    3cm piece of fresh ginger, peeled and thinly sliced

    1 tsp ground cumin

    1 tsp ground turmeric

    1 tsp ground coriander

    1–2 tbsp medium curry powder, to taste

    350g sweet potato, diced

    400g tin chopped tomatoes

    400ml full-fat coconut milk, plus extra if needed (optional)

    vegetable stock, as needed (optional)

    200g baby leaf spinach

    seasoning to taste

    cauliflower or broccoli rice (see page 146), or brown basmati
       rice, to serve

Heat the oil in a saucepan over a medium heat and add the onion, pepper, garlic, chillies and ginger. Combine well, then add the dried spices and sweet potato.

Cook for 5 minutes, then add the tomatoes and coconut milk.

Bring to the boil then reduce the heat to medium-low and cook for 10–15 minutes until the potato softens. You can add more liquid if needed (water, coconut milk or vegetable stock).

Add the spinach, and stir it into the curry until it has wilted and softened.

Season with salt and pepper to taste and serve with cauliflower rice.

Nutritional information per serving: 357 kcals, 22g fat, 31g net carbohydrates, 5.9g protein

Tofu and Pepper Wraps

Here is a perfectly quick-and-easy meal for busy evenings using my homemade and frozen harissa paste (or you can use bought harissa or fajita mix, if you prefer). A variety of healthy wraps is available from the supermarket today. I use gluten-free wraps made with quinoa and chia seeds. The tofu mixture can be made in advance and heated up just before serving. This dish can also be eaten cold for a quick lunch.

Serves 4

1 tbsp coconut oil or olive oil

400g firm organic tofu, cut into thick strips

1 red onion, sliced

1 red pepper, deseeded and sliced

1 green pepper, deseeded and sliced

2 tbsp Spicy Harissa Paste (see page 241) or fajita mix

4 tortilla wraps

60g rocket or peppery salad leaves

Heat the oil in a saucepan over a medium heat and cook the tofu, onion and pepper for 5–8 minutes or until the tofu is golden.

Add the harissa and combine well. Heat through. Fill the wraps with the tofu mix and a handful of rocket, and serve.

Nutritional information per serving 328 kcals, 15g fat, 24g net carbohydrates, 21g protein

Mushroom Cauliflower Risotto

This is a creamy rice-free risotto, made with cauliflower rice. You might be surprised by how great this tastes. It's very easy to prepare and is delicious topped with a sprinkle of chopped walnuts.

Serves 4

    10g dried porcini mushrooms

    300g cauliflower, cut into florets

    2 tsp coconut oil or olive oil

    1 onion, finely chopped

    400g mixed mushrooms (such as shiitake, oyster, chestnut, wild), chopped

    75ml white wine

    a handful of tarragon leaves, chopped

    zest of 1 lemon

    3 tbsp coconut cream

    a handful of parsley leaves, chopped

    30g walnuts, finely chopped

Soak the porcini mushrooms for 20 minutes or as directed on the pack. Drain through a sieve and leave to one side.

Meanwhile, put the cauliflower into a food processor or electric chopper and pulse for a few seconds until the cauliflower resembles rice. (If you don't have a processor you can grate the cauliflower, but it is messy and more time-consuming.) Leave to one side.

Heat the oil in a saucepan over a medium heat and cook the onion for 5–8 minutes until translucent. Add the fresh and dried mushrooms, and cook for a few minutes, stirring well.

Add the cauliflower rice and stir in, ensuring that it is completely covered in the oil mixture.

Add the wine and stir thoroughly. The wine will evaporate, but it will flavour the rice. Cook gently for 5–8 minutes until heated through and softened.

Add the tarragon and lemon zest. Stir in the coconut cream and heat through. Serve immediately, topped with the chopped parsley and walnuts.

Nutritional information per serving: 212 kcals, 12g fat, 16g net carbo-hydrates, 7.1g protein

Courgetti Vegan Bolognese

I think it is important to keep to traditional family favourites, especially when moving into a new diet, because food is not just about taste, it is also about satisfying the mind. If you are used to eating meat, you probably still want a similar feel and texture from some foods, but we want to do this without resorting to processed 'cheat meat' substitutes. This is my vegan version of a meaty bolognese.

■ Get ahead – this dish can be prepared in advance
■ Double up and freeze

Serves 6
    150g walnuts
    250g chestnut mushrooms
    1 tsp coconut oil or olive oil
    1 red onion, finely chopped
    2–3 garlic cloves, to taste, finely chopped
    1 red pepper, deseeded and finely chopped
    ½ (125g) aubergine, diced
    200ml vegetable stock or red wine
    400g tin chopped tomatoes

2 tbsp sun-dried tomato paste

60g red lentils

3 tsp Italian mixed herbs

1 tsp onion granules

ground black pepper

For the courgetti:

1 tsp coconut oil or olive oil.

3 courgettes, spiralised or cut into slithers using a vegetable
peeler (see tip on page 169)

Put the walnuts in a food processor or electric chopper and whizz until
they are chopped, but don't over-process them, you want to retain
texture, not create a paste.

Add the mushrooms to the food processor and give two short pulses
to chop them – again, do not over-process. The aim is to make a fine-
textured mixture similar to mince.

Heat the oil in a saucepan over a medium heat and cook the onion
for 5–8 minutes until soft and translucent. Add the garlic, pepper and
aubergine, and cook for another 2 minutes

Add the walnut mixture and cook for 5 minutes or until brown. Add
the stock and cook for 2 minutes, then add the tomatoes, tomato paste
and lentils. Stir well.

Add the mixed herbs and onion granules, and season with black
pepper. Bring to the boil, then reduce the heat and simmer very gently
for 15 minutes.

When almost ready to serve, make the courgetti. Heat the oil in a
saucepan over a medium heat and add the spiralised courgettes. Cook
for 3 minutes or until soft.

Serve the courgetti with the bolognese on top.

Nutritional information per serving 372 kcals, 27g fat, 17g net carbohydrates, 11g protein

Creamy Broccoli, Mushroom and Red Pepper Linguine

This recipe uses linguine, but you can use any spaghetti you like, ideally from a wheat-free source, for optimum health. I make this for my family using a wheat-free linguine, but as I no longer eat grains, I replace my portion with spiralised courgette or butternut squash.

Serves 4

  300g linguine, or courgettes or butternut squash, spiralised
    or cut into slithers using a vegetable peeler (see tip
    page 169)
  1 head of broccoli (about 300g), cut into florets
  1–2 tsp coconut oil or olive oil
  1 red onion, finely chopped
  3 garlic cloves, crushed
  100g button mushrooms, halved
  1 large red pepper, deseeded and diced
  5 tbsp coconut cream
  4 tbsp Vegan Parmesan (see page 237)
  a small handful of basil leaves, chopped

Cook the pasta, if using, in a saucepan of boiling water and cook for 9 minutes or according to the pack instructions. (If you are using spi-ralised vegetables, these will be cooked later.)

Meanwhile, put the broccoli in a steamer and steam over a high heat for 5 minutes until just tender but still with some bite.

Heat 1 tsp of the oil in saucepan over a medium heat and cook the onion, garlic, mushrooms and pepper for 5 minutes to soften.

Add the coconut cream, vegan Parmesan and basil. Combine well, then add the broccoli.

If serving with spiralised vegetables, when almost ready to serve, heat the remaining oil in a saucepan over a medium heat and add the spiralised courgettes. Cook for 2 minutes or until soft.

When the pasta is cooked, drain in a colander and tip into a large serving dish, or serve the vegetable spaghetti in the same way. Add the broccoli mixture and top with the basil, then serve.

Nutritional information per serving: 186 kcals, 9.4g fat, 11g net carbohydrates, 10g protein

Quick-and-Easy Aubergine and Tofu Curry

This curry can be made within 20 minutes, so it's perfect for a speedy workday evening meal. Serve with quinoa for extra protein, or you can use brown basmati rice – or, for an additional vegetable hit, opt for cauliflower or broccoli rice (see page 146).

Serves 4

1 tbsp coconut oil or olive oil

1 red onion, diced

2 garlic cloves, crushed

2 chillies, deseeded and finely chopped

3cm piece of fresh ginger, peeled and finely chopped

1 tbsp mild or medium curry powder

400g firm organic tofu, diced

2 aubergines, thickly diced

75g button mushrooms, halved

200ml coconut milk

250g chard, roughly chopped

a small handful of coriander leaves, chopped

seasoning to taste

30g flaked almonds

Heat the oil in a large saucepan over a medium heat and cook the onion, garlic, chillies and ginger for 2 minutes, then add the curry powder. Stir for 1 minute, then add the tofu, aubergines and mushrooms.

Continue to cook for 5–8 minutes until the tofu has browned and the vegetables are softened but not soggy.

Add the coconut milk, chard and coriander. Season well with salt and pepper to taste. Bring to the boil, then reduce the heat and simmer gently for 5 minutes. Serve sprinkled with the flaked almonds.

Nutritional information per serving: 374 kcals, 25g fat, 12g net carbo-hydrates, 21g protein

Weekend Meals

I t's time to kick back and relax at the weekend, but you might also have more time to spend creating some fantastic new dishes.

Look out for the recipes in this chapter that say 'Double up and freeze' or 'Get ahead'. These are also useful for weekday evening meals when planned in advance.

Baked Stuffed Aubergines

This is a great-tasting dish, which can be prepared in advance and left in the fridge until ready to bake. I top it with mixed nuts, but you can opt for seeds if you prefer. You can use the same filling recipe to stuff peppers, butternut squash or large beefeater tomatoes.

■ Get ahead – this dish can be prepared in advance

Serves 4

    2 aubergines, cut in half lengthways
    1 tbsp coconut oil, melted, or olive oil, plus extra for brushing
    1 red onion, diced

2 garlic cloves, crushed

1 red pepper, deseeded and diced

150g cherry tomatoes, halved

2 tbsp sun-dried tomato paste

1 tsp dried mixed herbs

60g oats

30g mixed nuts, chopped

seasoning to taste

80g baby leaf spinach

3–4 tbsp almond butter, melted

green salad, to serve

Preheat the oven to 180°C (160°C fan oven) Gas 4. Remove some of the flesh from the centre of the aubergine halves to enable them to be stuffed. Leave the flesh to one side.

Put the aubergines onto a baking tray, cut-side up. Brush the shells with a little coconut oil, then season with salt and pepper. Leave to rest.

Heat the oil in a saucepan over a medium heat and cook the onion, garlic and pepper for 5 minutes or until they start to soften.

Add the aubergine flesh, the tomatoes, tomato paste and herbs. Season with salt and pepper to taste. Cook for 5–10 minutes until softened.

Meanwhile, put the oats in a bowl and add the chopped nuts. Season and mix well.

Remove the saucepan from heat and stir in the spinach. Stuff the aubergines with the spinach mixture, then top with an even coating of oat mix.

Drizzle the almond nut butter over the oat mix, then cook in the oven for 15–20 minutes until golden. Serve with a lovely green salad.

Nutritional information per serving: 387 kcals, 26g fat, 22g net carbohydrates, 10g protein

Comforting Vegan Cottage Pie

When it comes to replicating a traditional meal with a vegan slant, this recipe ticks all the boxes. It's a nutrient-dense dish that will satisfy all the family, regardless of their dietary choices, and it will be just right for those who crave the food they grew up with while still enjoying a meat-free option. You can also plan ahead and make this in advance for a lovely evening meal for those crazy days when time is short.

■ Get ahead – this dish can be prepared in advance
■ Double up and freeze

Serves 6
    2 tsp coconut oil or olive oil
    1 large red onion, diced
    2 garlic cloves, finely chopped
    1 red pepper, deseeded and diced
    2 celery sticks, diced
    2 tsp coriander seeds, finely crushed
    300g chestnut mushrooms, finely chopped
    75g walnuts, finely chopped
    400g tin chopped tomatoes
    2 tbsp sun-dried tomato paste
    400g tin green lentils, drained and rinsed
    200ml vegetable stock
    1 tbsp vegan Worcester sauce
    2 tsp paprika
    1 tsp dried marjoram
    ½ tsp mixed herbs
    seasoning to taste
    steamed green vegetables, to serve

For the topping:

    1 butternut squash, cut into even-sized chunks
    800g sweet potatoes, cut into even-sized chunks
    2 garlic cloves, finely chopped
    1 red chilli (optional), deseeded and finely chopped
    3 tbsp coconut or olive oil

Put the butternut squash and sweet potato for the topping in a steamer and steam over a high heat for 15 minutes or until soft. Leave to one side.

Meanwhile, make the mince mixture. Heat the oil in a large saucepan over a medium heat and cook the onion, garlic, pepper and celery for 1 minute, then add the crushed coriander seeds.

Add the mushrooms and walnuts, and cook for 5 minutes or until the mushrooms start to soften.

Add the remaining ingredients, then bring to the boil, reduce the heat and simmer for 10 minutes. Season to taste. Preheat the oven to 180°C (160°C fan oven) Gas 4.

To make the topping, put the butternut squash and sweet potato into a large bowl or the drained pan of your steamer. Add the garlic, chilli, if using, and the oil. Mash well, then season to taste.

Put the vegetable base into the ovenproof dish and spoon on the topping. Spread out evenly using a fork. (You can cool and freeze the cottage pie at this stage or store it in the fridge until ready to cook, if you like.) Cook in the oven for 25 minutes. Serve with green vegetables.

Nutritional information per serving 470 kcals, 21g fat, 52g net carbohydrates, 14g protein

Beetroot Risotto

This vibrant red risotto looks dramatic, especially topped with dark green salad leaves, such as rocket, to emphasise the fabulous colour. The rice is quick to cook, but as the beetroot is roasted, you could roast it in advance if you want to speed up the process.

Serves 4

500g raw beetroot, peeled and cut into thick chunks
1 tbsp olive oil
1 tsp coconut oil or olive oil
1 red onion, finely chopped
2 garlic cloves, crushed
600ml hot stock
300g Arborio or other risotto rice
200ml red wine
3 tbsp coconut cream (optional)
salt and ground black pepper

Preheat the oven to 180°C (160°C fan oven) Gas 4. Put the beetroot into a roasting tin and drizzle over the olive oil, shake well to distribute the oil then roast for 20 minutes.

Heat the teaspoon of coconut oil or olive oil in a large saucepan over a medium heat and cook the onion and garlic for 5–8 minutes until translucent. Add the roasted beetroot and stir well. Keep the stock simmering on the hob.

Reduce the heat for the beetroot mixture to medium-low, then add the rice and stir in, ensuring that it is completely covered in the oil mixture. Don't allow the rice to stick to the pan!

Add the wine and stir thoroughly. The wine will evaporate, but it will flavour the rice.

Add a ladleful of the hot stock and stir until absorbed into the rice.

Repeat with the remaining stock – always waiting until the stock has been absorbed before adding more.

After 12–15 minutes the rice should be tender but still with some bite. If you would like a creamy risotto, stir in the coconut cream. Season to taste and serve immediately.

Nutritional information per serving: 429 kcals, 5.9g fat, 74g net carbohydrates, 8.4g protein

Loaded Roasted Brussels Sprouts

Brussels sprouts aren't just for Christmas! They are really delicious roasted at any time of the year – and even in salads as well. A great source of vitamins B_6, C and K, Brussels sprouts also contain manganese and folate, as well as fibre. Serve this dish as a main meal, or omit the tofu and walnuts, and serve it as a side dish.

Serves 4
  400g Brussels sprouts
  3 garlic cloves, roughly chopped
  2 red chillies, deseeded and roughly
    chopped
  1 red onion, cut into wedges
  2 rosemary sprigs
  2 thyme sprigs
  3 tbsp coconut oil, melted
  400g organic tempeh or tofu, cut
    into chunks
  75g walnuts, roughly chopped
  3 tomatoes, chopped
  seasoning to taste

Preheat the oven to 180°C (160°C fan oven) Gas 4. Put the Brussels sprouts in a roasting tin and add the garlic, chillies, onion, rosemary and thyme. Drizzle over 2 tbsp of the oil and combine well, ensuring it is all covered. Roast for 30–40 minutes until tender.

Meanwhile, heat the remaining coconut oil in a saucepan over a medium heat and cook the tempeh until browned. Remove from heat and put to one side.

Remove the Brussels sprout mix from the oven and tip it into a large serving dish. Stir in the tempeh, walnuts and tomatoes, and combine well. Season to taste before serving.

Nutritional information per serving: 462 kcals, 32g fat, 14g net carbohydrates, 24g protein

Vegan 'Meaty' Lasagne

This is as near as I can get to a traditional lasagne, but without meat and dairy. I have used butternut squash lasagne sheets (which are now available in most large supermarkets) instead of lasagne sheets, but this is entirely your choice. Sheets of courgette also work well. Both the components of the lasagne can be made in advance and stored in the fridge. Alternatively, you can freeze the lasagne.

- Get ahead – this dish can be prepared in advance
- Double up and freeze

Serves 6
    150g walnuts
    250g mushrooms
    1 tsp coconut oil
    1 red onion, finely chopped

2–3 garlic cloves, to taste, crushed

1 red pepper, deseeded and finely chopped

200ml vegetable stock, red wine or water

400g tin chopped tomatoes

1 tbsp sun-dried tomato paste

50g red lentils

2 tsp dried Italian or mixed herbs

½ tsp dried basil

black pepper to taste

400g butternut squash lasagne sheets

green salad, to serve

For the sauce:

3 tbsp olive oil

2 tbsp cornflour

400ml unsweetened almond milk or other plant-based milk

4 tbsp nutritional yeast flakes

1 tsp onion granules

1 tsp mustard

seasoning to taste

Put the walnuts in a food processor or electric chopper and whizz until they are chopped, but don't over-process them, you want to retain texture, not create a paste.

Add the mushrooms to the food processor and give two short pulses to chop them – again, do not over-process. The aim is to make a fine-textured mixture similar to mince.

Heat the oil in a saucepan over a medium heat and cook the onion for 5–8 minutes until soft and translucent. Add the garlic and pepper, and cook for 2 minutes.

Add walnut mixture and cook for 5 minutes or until brown. Add the stock and cook for 2 minutes, then add the tomatoes, tomato paste and lentils. Stir well.

Add the herbs and season with pepper. Bring to the boil, then reduce the heat and simmer very gently for 15 minutes. Preheat the oven to 170°C (150°C fan oven) Gas 3.

Meanwhile, to make the sauce, heat the oil in a saucepan over a medium-low heat and stir in the cornflour until it forms a paste. Gradually add the almond milk, stirring continuously. I use a balloon whisk, as I find it helps to prevent lumps. Once you have a nice smooth sauce, add the nutritional yeast flakes, onion granules and mustard. Season to taste.

Put some of the mince mixture on the base of a lasagne dish or shallow ovenproof dish around 20cm. Top with the butternut squash sheets, followed by a layer of the sauce. Repeat the layers, finishing with the sauce.

Cook in the oven for 20 minutes or until golden and bubbling. Serve with a green salad.

Nutritional information per serving: 435 kcals, 30g fat, 23g net carbohydrates, 13g protein

Simply the Best Nut Roast

This is a fantastic recipe for a roast or Christmas dinner, and it is always popular with meat eaters and vegetarians. It really does speed up the preparation process if you can use a food processor to chop the nuts.

■ Get ahead – this dish can be prepared in advance
■ Double up and freeze

Serves 6
   2 tsp coconut oil or olive oil
   1 red onion, finely chopped

2 garlic cloves, crushed
150g Brazil nuts, finely chopped
150g cashew nuts, finely chopped
250g mushrooms, finely chopped
2 tsp yeast extract
1 tsp dried thyme
1 tsp Italian or mixed herbs
25g ground almonds or coconut flour
seasoning to taste

Preheat the oven to 190°C (170°C fan oven) Gas 5 and line a 900g loaf tin with baking parchment. Heat the oil in a saucepan over a medium heat and cook the onion and garlic for 5–8 minutes until translucent.

Add the chopped nuts and mushrooms and cook for 5 minutes. Add the yeast extract, herbs and ground almonds. Season to taste.

Transfer to the prepared loaf tin and press down firmly. Bake for 40 minutes or until golden on top. The uncooked mixture can be frozen.

Nutritional information per serving: 396 kcals, 32.8g fat, 9.5g net carbohydrates, 12.5g protein

Black-Eyed Bean Chilli

You can use any beans for this punchy chilli, or even a mixed bean combination. Like any chilli, this tastes even better when cooked the day before.

- Get ahead – this dish can be prepared in advance
- Double up and freeze

Serves 4

- 1 tsp coconut oil or olive oil
- 1 large red onion, chopped
- 2 star anise
- 2 garlic cloves, crushed
- 1 carrot, finely diced
- 1 red pepper, deseeded and diced
- 1 celery stick, diced
- 1–2 red chillies, to taste, deseeded and finely chopped
- 1 tsp marjoram
- 2 tsp dried oregano
- 1–2 tsp chilli powder, to taste
- 2 tsp smoked paprika
- ½ tsp cayenne pepper
- 400g tinned chopped tomatoes
- 2 tbsp sun-dried tomato paste
- 400g tin black-eyed beans, drained and rinsed
- 75g red lentils
- 350ml water or vegetable stock
- brown basmati rice, or for less carbs, cauliflower rice and coconut yogurt, to serve

Heat the oil in a saucepan over a medium heat, add the onion and star anise and cook for 3 minutes. Add the garlic, carrot, pepper, celery and chillies and cook for 5–8 minutes or until they start to soften slightly. Remove the star anise.

Add the herbs and dried spices, then the tomatoes, tomato paste, beans and lentils. Cook for 1 minute, then add the water or stock and stir well. Bring to the boil, then reduce the heat and simmer over a low heat for 25 minutes, stirring occasionally. Serve with rice and a dollop of coconut yogurt.

Nutritional information per serving: 382 kcals, 13g fat, 43g net carbohydrates, 17g protein

Vegetable and Chickpea Casserole

This is a simple recipe but great for those colder evenings when you
crave comfort food.

■ Get ahead – this dish can be prepared in advance
■ Double up and freeze

Serves 6

2 tsp coconut oil or olive oil

1 red onion, sliced

1–2 garlic cloves, to taste, crushed

1–2 chillies, to taste, deseeded (optional)

1 red pepper, deseeded and sliced

2 celery sticks, sliced

1 sweet potato, diced

1 carrot, sliced

1 courgette, sliced

400g tin chopped tomatoes

2 tsp fresh oregano or 1 tsp dried

½ tsp dried marjoram

½ tsp dried tarragon

3 tsp thyme leaves or 1 tsp dried thyme

1 tbsp chopped parsley leaves

2 tbsp nutritional yeast flakes

400g tin chickpeas, drained and rinsed

75g red lentils

350ml vegetable stock, plus extra if needed

1 bay leaf
steamed green vegetables, to serve
salt and ground black pepper

Heat the oil in a large saucepan over a medium heat and cook the onion and garlic for 5 minutes or until they start to soften.

Add chillies, pepper, celery, sweet potato, carrot and courgette, and cook for 3 minutes, stirring well to prevent sticking.

Add the remaining ingredients, bring to the boil, then reduce the heat and simmer for 30 minutes.

Check the mixture halfway through to ensure that there is enough liquid and add more stock if necessary. Season to taste with salt and pepper. Serve with green vegetables.

Nutritional information per serving 210 kcals, 3.6g fat, 30g net carbohydrates, 10g protein

Sweet Potato and Chickpea Curry

This dish looks amazing when served with broccoli rice – the green contrasts well against the orange of the curry, and the nutty flavour of the broccoli really complements the flavours. (Top with some almond flakes and a garnish of coriander leaves.)

■ Get ahead – this dish can be prepared in advance
■ Double up and freeze

Serves 6
    2 tsp coconut oil
    1 large red onion, diced
    2 garlic cloves, crushed

3cm piece of fresh ginger, peeled and finely chopped

1–2 red chillies, to taste, deseeded and finely chopped

½ red pepper, deseeded and chopped

1 tsp cumin seeds

2 tbsp medium curry powder

1 tsp ground turmeric

3 sweet potatoes, cubed

2 bay leaves

400ml tin full-fat coconut milk

400g tin chopped tomatoes

400g tin chickpeas, drained and rinsed

juice of 1 lemon

80g baby leaf spinach

a small handful of coriander leaves

salt and ground black pepper

coriander leaves and a small handful of almond flakes,
    to garnish

broccoli rice (see page 146), quinoa or brown basmati
    rice, to serve

Heat the oil in a large saucepan over a medium heat and cook the onion, garlic, ginger, chillies and pepper for 2 minutes.

Add the dried spices and combine well for 1 minute. Add the sweet potatoes and bay leaves, and cook for 2 minutes.

Add the remaining ingredients, except the spinach and coriander leaves, and season with salt and pepper. Bring to the boil then reduce the heat and simmer for 20 minutes. Check occasionally and stir to ensure that it doesn't stick to the base of the pan. Add some water if you feel it needs more liquid. Garnish with coriander leaves and flaked almonds and serve with broccoli rice.

Nutritional information per serving: 335 kcals, 16g fat, 38g net carbohydrates, 6.8g protein

Vegan Celebration Pie

Packed full of goodness from the vegetables, nuts and lentils, this pie is wholesome and filling, with a pastry base and a crispy topping. You can prepare the pie in advance, so it's ideal for dinner parties. Serve it with salads on a summer's day or steamed green vegetables, new potatoes and a vegetable gravy for a warming winter meal.

■ Get ahead – this dish can be prepared in advance
■ Double up and freeze

Serves 8

250g buckwheat or spelt flour, plus extra for dusting
125g coconut oil, chilled and cut into small pieces, plus extra
    for greasing
200g Puy lentils
1 tsp coconut oil or olive oil
1 large red onion, diced
2 garlic cloves, crushed
175g chestnut mushrooms, finely chopped
175g cashew nuts, finely chopped
80g baby leaf spinach
1 tsp soy sauce or coconut aminos
1 tsp yeast extract
1 tsp mixed herbs
1 tsp dried marjoram
1 tsp onion granules
seasoning to taste
green salad, to serve

For the topping:
3 tbsp nutritional yeast flakes

75g spelt or buckwheat breadcrumbs

a small handful of parsley leaves, chopped

Put the flour in a food processor and add the chilled coconut oil. Whizz until the mix resembles breadcrumbs. (Alternatively, rub the coconut oil gently into the flour using your fingers, but try not to handle the mixture too much.)

Add 3–5 tbsp cold water, a little at a time, and mix with a fork until it comes together. Use your hands to form a dough. Wrap the dough in cling film and put it in the fridge to rest for 30 minutes or until needed.

Cook the Puy lentils in a saucepan of boiling water for 15 minutes or until they are soft but still retain the nutty bite.

Meanwhile, heat the 1 tsp oil in a saucepan over a medium heat and cook the onion and garlic for 2 minutes. Add the mushrooms and cashew nuts, and cook for 4 minutes, then add the spinach, a little at a time until it reduces into the mixture.

Add the soy sauce, yeast extract, herbs, onion granules and 150ml water.

Drain the lentils and add them to the mixture. Cook for 5 minutes over a low heat. Season to taste. Leave the mixture to cool. Preheat the oven to 180°C (160°C fan oven) Gas 4 and grease a 23cm pie dish.

Roll out the pasty on a lightly floured work surface to a little larger than the pie dish. Put into the dish and press down lightly. Flatten the edge to the flat edge of the dish and trim to neaten.

Fill the pastry case with the mushroom filling and level the mixture to form a flat top.

To make the topping, mix the nutritional yeast flakes with the bread-crumbs and parsley, season with salt and pepper and sprinkle over the top of the pie. Bake for 25–35 minutes or until golden. Serve with a green salad.

Nutritional information per serving: 492 kcals, 28g fat, 41g net carbo-hydrates, 15g protein

Pumpkin Stuffed with Quinoa and Fennel

You can use a large butternut squash or any other squash if you can't get small pumpkins. This recipe uses my olive tapenade to enrich the flavour of the fennel and butter bean filling. This recipe can be prepared in advance and just popped into the oven when ready to cook.

Serves 4

1 small pumpkin or squash (about 300g), left whole
2 tbsp coconut oil, melted, or olive oil
100g quinoa, rinsed (see page 149)
1 red onion, diced
2 garlic cloves, crushed
1 fennel bulb, diced
1 courgette, diced
2 tbsp Olive Tapenade (page 243)
200g tinned butter beans, drained and rinsed
50g baby leaf spinach, roughly chopped
50g walnuts, roughly chopped
seasoning to taste
green salad, to serve

Preheat the oven to 180°C (160°C fan oven) Gas 4. Cut the top off the pumpkin and retain it to use as a lid when serving, if you wish.

Carefully scoop out the seeds and pith, and discard. Brush with a little of the coconut oil. Put in a baking sheet and roast for 30 minutes.

Meanwhile, put the quinoa in a saucepan and add 250ml water. Bring to the boil then reduce the heat and cook for 10–15 minutes or until the grains have swollen.

Drain in a sieve and leave to one side.

Heat the remaining oil in a saucepan over a medium heat and cook the onion and garlic, fennel and courgette for 5 minutes to soften.

Add the tapenade, quinoa, butter beans, spinach and walnuts, and combine well. Cook for 5 minutes, then season to taste.

Fill the pumpkin with the quinoa mixture, add the top, if using, then return it to the oven and bake for 10 minutes. Serve the stuffed pumpkin cut into wedges with a green salad.

Nutritional information per serving: 349kcals, 19.8g fat, 26.6g net carbohydrates, 12.4g protein

Variation: You could also use this filling to stuff portobello mushrooms. Cook them for 15 minutes at 180°C (160°C fan oven) Gas 4.

Green Bean and Tomato Bredie

A bredie is a South African stew, and this is my take on a vegan version. You can serve this with rice or quinoa or with some flatbreads topped with hummus.

■ Get ahead – this dish can be prepared in advance
■ Double up and freeze

Serves 4
   2 tsp coconut oil or olive oil
   1 large red onion, chopped
   2 garlic cloves, chopped
   3cm piece of fresh ginger, peeled and finely grated
   1 red chilli, deseeded and finely chopped
   1 carrot, diced
   2 sweet potatoes, cut into chunks
   1 tsp chopped rosemary leaves or ½ tsp dried rosemary
   400g tin chopped tomatoes

200ml vegetable stock or water

1 tbsp coconut aminos or soy sauce

200g green beans, each cut into 2 or 3 pieces

75g Swiss chard or kale leaves, torn into a few pieces

a small handful of coriander leaves, chopped

rice or quinoa, or spelt, buckwheat or low-carb, grain-free
   flatbreads topped with hummus, to serve

Heat the oil in a saucepan over a medium heat and cook the onion, garlic, ginger and chilli for 5–8 minutes until the onion starts to become translucent.

Add the carrot and the sweet potatoes, and cook for 5 minutes, stirring constantly.

Add the rosemary, tomatoes, stock, coconut aminos or soy sauce. Bring to the boil, then reduce the heat and simmer for 15 minutes, stirring occasionally.

Add the green beans, chard and coriander, and cook for a further 10 minutes or until the vegetables are tender and the liquid has reduced. Serve with rice or flatbreads topped with hummus.

Nutritional information per serving: 205 kcals, 3.3g fat, 35g net carbohydrates, 4.8g protein

Pesto and Avocado Pizza

This really is richly flavoured and bursting with nutrients. If you don't want the heat of my homemade chilli-flavoured pesto, you could use your own milder green vegan version. My standard buckwheat base can be made in advance.

■ Get ahead – this dish can be prepared in advance

Makes 8 Slices

    175g buckwheat flour, plus extra for dusting

    ½ tsp baking powder

    ¼ tsp chilli powder (optional)

    20g chia seeds

    ½ tsp dried herbes de Provence or Italian herbs

For the topping

    3 tbsp Chilli and Coriander Pesto (page 240)

    4 spring onions, finely chopped

    ½ green pepper, deseeded and sliced

    40g pitted green olives, halved

    1 ripe avocado, flesh scooped from the skin and sliced

    a small handful of rocket

    a small handful of baby leaf spinach

    olive oil or avocado oil, for drizzling

Sift the buckwheat flour with the baking powder and chilli powder, if using, into a bowl. Tip in any bran remaining in the sieve. Add the chia seeds and herbs. Combine well, then add 200ml cold water, a little at a time, and stir well using a fork to form a dough. Leave for 5 minutes, then use your hands to form the dough into a ball. You may need to add more water if it is too dry. Preheat the oven to 180°C (160°C fan oven) Gas 4, or your standard pizza setting.

Knead the dough on a lightly floured work surface for 5 minutes. Add a little more flour if it is too sticky, or a little more water if too dry.

Roll it out gently to form a circle about 22cm in diameter and put it onto a baking sheet. Bake for 10 minutes.

Spread the base with pesto, then add the spring onions, pepper and olives. Return the pizza to the oven for a further 10 minutes.

Put the avocado, rocket and spinach on top of the hot pizza. Drizzle with some olive oil and serve immediately.

Nutritional information per slice: 315kcals, 13.8g fat, 34g net carbohydrates, 9g protein

Making the dough in advance: The dough can be kept in the fridge for up to 24 hours. Alternatively, you can freeze the rolled-out pizza base between sheets of baking parchment. If you make more than one base at a time for freezing, separate each with a sheet of baking parchment.

Spicy Tofu Burgers

Traditional burgers are always popular and are quick to prepare. These vegan burgers follow the trend and can be served with a burger bun – buckwheat baps taste great – or a salad. The burgers can be grilled, fried or baked and are a healthy barbecue option.

- Get ahead – this dish can be prepared in advance
- Double up and freeze

Serves 6

    400g tin chickpeas, drained and rinsed
    400g pack firm organic tofu
    1–2 tbsp unsweetened almond milk or other plant-based
       milk, if needed
    1 tsp coconut oil or olive oil, plus extra for shallow frying (optional)
    1 red onion, finely chopped
    1–2 garlic cloves, to taste, crushed
    1 red chilli, deseeded and finely chopped
    1 celery stick, finely chopped
    1 tbsp sun-dried tomato paste
    1–3 tsp garam masala, to taste
    a splash of soy sauce or coconut aminos

2 tsp finely chopped fresh parsley

seasoning to taste

2–4 tbsp fine polenta, as needed

spelt or buckwheat baps and salad, to serve

Put the chickpeas in a large bowl and mash until soft. Add tofu and continue to mash until mixed thoroughly. You may need to add a little milk to encourage the mixture to form a good mash – don't overdo this though.

Heat the coconut oil in a saucepan over a medium heat and cook the onion, garlic, chilli and celery for 5–8 minutes until soft.

Add the onion mixture to the chickpea mixture. Add the sun-dried tomato paste, garam masala, soy sauce and parsley. Season and combine well.

Add the polenta, a little at a time, stirring to incorporate it well. You might not need it all – it is only used to help the mixture form into balls.

Mix thoroughly and form into 6 balls – these should be firm but moist. Use the palm of your hand to flatten the balls into burger shapes.

Grill, or fry the burgers in coconut oil, for 5 minutes on both sides or until golden.

Serve in a bap garnished with salad.

Nutritional information per serving: 214 kcals, 10g fat, 14g net carbohydrates, 14g protein

Oven cooking and freezing burgers

Oven cooking: You can also oven cook the burgers at 180°C (160°C fan oven) Gas 4 for 20 minutes.

Freezing: It's worth making a double batch of these burgers and freezing them. Remember to use small squares of baking parchment to separate each burger before freezing to prevent them from sticking together.

Nut and Mushroom Balls

With a base of chickpeas, these tasty balls are nourishing and filling. I like to serve them with a tomato sauce and vegetable pasta. They can take a little while to prepare, but as they freeze, it's worth making double the amount so that you have a speedy meal for another day as well.

- Get ahead – this dish can be prepared in advance
- Double up and freeze

Serves 6

150g mushrooms
1 large red onion, cut into quarters
125g walnuts
2 tbsp flaxseeds
1 tbsp chia seeds
1 tsp coconut oil or olive oil, plus extra for shallow frying
2 garlic cloves, crushed
400g tin chickpeas, drained and rinsed
1 tsp dried oregano
1 tsp dried marjoram
2 tsp paprika
3 tbsp oats
2 tsp vegan Worcester sauce or coconut aminos
2 tbsp sun-dried tomato paste
Tomato Sauce (page 245) and spiralised courgette,
   to serve

Put the mushrooms, onion and walnuts in a food processor or electric chopper. Blitz them until finely chopped – don't over-process or the mixture will become mushy. (Alternatively, finely chop them.)

Put the flaxseeds and chia seeds in a bowl and add 100ml water. Leave to one side.

Heat the oil in a saucepan over a medium heat, add the garlic and the mushroom mixture and cook for 5 minutes.

Add the chickpeas, herbs, paprika, oats, Worcester sauce and tomato paste, and combine well.

Transfer to a bowl and add the flax mixture. Combine well and leave for a few minutes to rest.

Form into golf-ball-sized balls, and put them on a piece of baking parchment. Heat a little oil in a frying pan and fry the balls on all sides for 8–10 minutes or until golden. Alternatively, preheat the oven to 180°C (160°C fan oven) Gas 4 and oven cook for 15 minutes. Serve with a tomato sauce and spiralised courgette.

Nutritional information per serving: 334 kcals, 25g fat, 15g net carbohydrates, 9.6g protein

Freezing: To freeze, pop on a baking tray lined with baking parchment, ensuring the balls are not touching each other. Freeze, then remove the balls and put into freezer bags, then return them to the freezer.

Moroccan-Style Vegetable Tagine

Make this wholesome vegetable version of the traditional Moroccan dish flavoured with harissa. Serve it with quinoa, as this is nutritionally preferable to the traditional couscous.

- Get ahead – this dish can be prepared in advance
- Double up and freeze

Serves 6

2 tsp coconut oil or olive oil

1 red onion, diced

2–3 garlic cloves, to taste, roughly chopped

1 red chilli, finely chopped

2cm piece of fresh ginger, peeled and finely chopped

1 red or yellow pepper, deseeded and diced

1 carrot, diced

1 sweet potato, peeled and diced

1 courgette, thickly diced

1 aubergine, thickly diced

1–2 tsp chilli powder, to taste

½ tsp chilli flakes (optional)

2 tsp Spicy Harissa Paste (page 241)

1 tsp ground turmeric

1 tsp ground cinnamon

½ tsp ground coriander

2 tsp finely chopped mint leaves or ½ tsp dried mint

400g tin chopped tomatoes

75g red lentils

400g tin chickpeas, drained and rinsed

40g dried ready-to-eat apricots (optional), halved

450ml vegetable stock or water, plus extra if needed

a small handful of coriander leaves, chopped

30g flaked almonds

quinoa, to serve

Heat the oil in a large saucepan and cook the onion, garlic, chilli and ginger for 1 minute.

Add the pepper, carrot, sweet potato, courgette and aubergine, and cook for 5 minutes, then add the harissa paste and spices. Stir over the heat for 30 seconds or until the spices release their flavour.

Add the mint, tomatoes, lentils, chickpeas and apricots, if using. Add the stock. Bring to the boil, then reduce the heat and simmer for 20–30 minutes until the vegetables are tender. Add more stock if needed. Top with the chopped coriander and flaked almonds, and serve with quinoa.

Nutritional information per serving: 254 kcals, 5.8g fat, 34g net carbohydrates, 11g protein

Slow cooking: This recipe can also be made in the slow cooker. Put all the ingredients into the slow cooker and cook on low for 6 hours.

Vegetable Biryani

This filling dish can be eaten on its own or made as part of a selection of Indian dishes to serve at a dinner party. A good spread could include the Aubergine and Tofu Curry, Sweet Potato and Spinach Curry and the Creamy Masoor Dhal.

▓ Get ahead – this dish can be prepared in advance

Serves 6
    1 tsp coconut oil or olive oil
    1 red onion, finely chopped
    2–3 garlic cloves, to taste, crushed
    2 red chillies, deseeded and finely chopped
    2cm piece of fresh ginger, peeled and grated
    1 tsp cumin seeds
    2 tsp mustard seeds
    1 tsp ground coriander
    1 tsp chilli powder
    1 tsp ground turmeric

1 aubergine, diced

1 courgette, diced

1 red pepper, deseeded and diced

2 tomatoes, diced

3 tbsp coconut cream

400g basmati rice

1 litre vegetable stock

chopped coriander leaves, to garnish

Preheat the oven to 190°C (170°C fan oven) Gas 5. Heat the coconut oil in a saucepan over a medium heat and cook the onion, garlic, chillies and ginger for 2–3 minutes. Add the dried spices, the vegetables and tomatoes. Stir and cook for 5 minutes to help soften.

Add the coconut cream and stir well. Remove from the heat. Tip the dry basmati rice into the pan with the vegetables and mix well, then transfer to a large ovenproof dish.

Pour over the stock, then cover with foil. (If cooking in advance you can cool it and store it in the fridge at this stage.) Cook in the oven for 30–40 minutes until the rice is tender. Garnish with coriander and serve.

Nutritional information per serving 330 kcals, 4.4g fat, 61g net carbohydrates, 7.6g protein

Quick Desserts

Who doesn't love a dessert occasionally? This chapter is all about having delicious and satisfying desserts that avoid dairy – and also steer clear of sugar. I do find it frustrating when vegan cakes, sweets and desserts are laden with dried fruit and maple syrup, as if these natural sources of sugar are somehow less bothersome to our bodies. Sadly, they are not, but these sugar-free desserts contain healthy and satisfying ingredients, and you can enjoy them when you need a treat.

Chocolate Mousse

My chocolate mousse tastes luxurious and is also rich in essential fatty acids – perfect!

Serves 2

    1 ripe avocado, flesh scooped from the skin

    2 tbsp cacao or unsweetened cocoa powder

    75–125ml unsweetened almond milk or other plant-based milk

    2 tsp rice malt syrup, or to taste, or stevia drops, to taste

    berries, to serve

Optional extras (choose one):
   a few drops to taste of either vanilla, orange or mint extract
   1–2 tsp peanut butter, to taste
   4 hazelnuts

Put the avocado and cacao into a blender or food processor and add 75ml milk. Whizz until smooth. Add more liquid until you get your desired consistency.

Taste and add sweetener to taste. If you like, add one of the optional extras to the mix and whizz to combine. Pour into two individual ramekins and chill in the fridge until firm. Serve with berries.

Nutritional information per serving: 243 kcals, 19.2g fat, 6.5g net carbohydrates, 6.6g protein

Variation: If you would like a creamier mousse, stir in 4–5 tbsp coconut cream. This also removes some of the bitterness from the chocolate and is recommended if you are not accustomed to rich, dark chocolate.

Raspberry Panna Cotta

Vegans don't eat anything with gelatine in it, which can rule out some of the standard desserts; however, agar agar is a good vegan replacement and can work well. Frozen, rather than fresh, raspberries work particularly well here because they create more of a sauce in the base of the panna cotta – but both taste great.

Serves 4
   100g fresh or frozen raspberries, plus extra to serve
   1 tsp vanilla bean paste, or 2 vanilla pods
   400ml coconut milk or unsweetened plant-based milk

100g coconut cream

2 tbsp natural sweetener such as erythritol or xylitol, or stevia
drops, to taste

2 tsp agar agar flakes

sprigs of mint to decorate

Crush the raspberries and divide among six serving glasses. If using vanilla pods, cut the pods in half horizontally and scrape out the seeds onto a plate.

Put the milk in a saucepan and add the coconut cream, the vanilla bean paste or vanilla seeds and the sweetener. Heat over a medium heat and bring almost to a simmer.

Add the agar agar flakes and, using a balloon whisk, whisk thoroughly until they are completely dissolved.

Pour the mixture very carefully over the raspberries. Chill the glasses in the fridge for 3–4 hours or until set. Serve with the remaining raspberries and a sprig of mint to decorate. The dessert can be stored in the fridge for up to 3 days.

Nutritional information per serving 302 kcals, 27g fat, 12g net carbohydrates, 2.5g protein

Dark Chocolate Pecan Tart

The combination of sweet pecan nuts against the rich chocolate is divine. I like to serve this with some sliced strawberries and a dollop of coconut cream or coconut yogurt.

Serves 10

300g pecan nuts

3 tbsp coconut oil, melted, plus extra for greasing

400ml coconut milk or other unsweetened plant-based milk

2 tbsp cornflour

250g dark, vegan chocolate (minimum 85% cocoa solids),
    broken into pieces

1 shot of espresso

1 tsp vanilla paste

4 tbsp xylitol or erythritol, or stevia drops, to taste

strawberries, to decorate

Put the pecan nuts in a food processor and blitz until they resemble breadcrumbs.

Tip into a bowl and add the melted coconut oil. Combine well.

Grease a 20cm flan tin thoroughly with coconut oil.

Put the crumbled pecan nuts into the tin and spread them out. Press them down to form a solid base, then put the tin in the fridge to chill for 20 minutes.

Reserve 2 tbsp of the milk and pour the remainder into a saucepan over a medium heat. Bring the milk to a mild simmer, then reduce the heat to medium-low.

Put the cornflour in a bowl and mix with the reserved milk to form a liquid paste.

Put the chocolate in the hot milk and add the espresso, vanilla and sweetener. Leave to melt, stirring occasionally.

Add the cornflour mixture and stir in, then take a balloon whisk, and whisk to remove any lumps until the mixture is thick and glossy. Pour onto the nut base and chill in the fridge overnight, or for at least 3 hours, until set. Add a few strawberries to decorate, and serve. The dessert can be stored in the fridge for up to 3 days.

Nutritional information per serving: 499 kcals, 45g fat, 20g net carbohydrates, 6.3g protein

Baked Cinnamon Apples

Here is a traditional autumnal treat that is effortless to produce. I would advise to always use Bramley apples, as they are the best cooking apples for flavour and texture when cooked.

Serves 4

    4 Bramley apples, cored but not peeled

    40g hazelnuts

    40g pecan nuts

    2 tbsp coconut oil

    2 tsp rice malt syrup, Sukrin Fibre Syrup or xylitol

    2 tsp ground cinnamon

    coconut yogurt or vegan ice cream, to serve

Preheat the oven to 180°C (160°C fan oven) Gas 4. Put the apples in an ovenproof dish.

Put the nuts in a food processor and whizz until they resemble breadcrumbs. Add the coconut oil, rice malt syrup and cinnamon, and process until it forms a thick paste.

Fill the centre of each apple with the nut mixture, then bake in the oven for 20–30 minutes until soft. Serve with some coconut yogurt or ice cream.

Nutritional information per serving: 270 kcals, 21g fat, 16g net carbohydrates, 3.2g protein

Variation: You can also stuff the apples with my Cinnamon and Apple Granola (page 94).

Fruit Crumble Mug

This recipe was created because my son loves fruit crumbles and pies. Because I tend to prefer berries and yogurt, it was a waste in our house to make a large crumble. This individual crumble is simple and satisfying.

I am a big fan of frozen fruit. In the autumn I store up the apples, chop and freeze them ready for a quick meal, and I always have frozen berries in my freezer to add colour and flavour. You can use fresh or frozen fruit in this recipe. My sugar-free granola is always on hand, so combining this with the fruit makes a very easy dessert.

Serves 1
    ½ mug of frozen berries or use any prepared fruit, including
        diced apple
    xylitol, erythritol, or stevia drops, to taste
    a pinch of ground cinnamon or grated nutmeg, or some berries
        (if using apple – optional)
    20g Cinnamon Apple Granola (see page 94)
    coconut yogurt, to serve

Put the berries in a saucepan and add 1 tbsp water; if you are using hard fruit, add 3 tbsp water. Cook over a medium heat for 2 minutes for berries and 5 minutes for hard fruits, or until softened. (Alternatively, cook for a few minutes in the microwave on full power.)

Stir in the sweetener to taste. If you are cooking apple, you might want to add the cinnamon or nutmeg, or a few frozen berries.

Once the fruit is cooked, transfer it to a mug and top with the granola. Serve with a dollop of coconut yogurt.

Nutritional information per serving: 190 kcals, 11.3g fat, 13.7g net carbohydrates, 4.6g protein

Peach and Raspberry Bakes

Make this dessert in the summer when peaches are in season and at their ripest and sweetest. Baking the peaches releases their sweetness, so I don't need to add any sweetener, but if you feel it is needed, you could drizzle a little Sukrin Fibre, rice malt syrup or stevia liquid onto the peaches before baking them. You could also add a few drops of vanilla stevia liquid to the coconut cream, if you like it very sweet.

Serves 4

4 ripe peaches, halved and stoned
100g fresh or frozen raspberries
60g flaked almonds

For the topping

200ml coconut cream or coconut yogurt
1 tsp vanilla extract
zest of 1 orange

Preheat the oven to 170°C (150°C fan oven) Gas 3. Put the peaches on a baking tray, cut-side upwards.

Put the raspberries in the stone cavity of each peach half. Sprinkle the flaked almonds over the top, retaining a few for later. Bake for 15 minutes.

Meanwhile, to make the topping, mix the coconut cream with the vanilla and orange zest.

When the peaches are ready, put them in individual serving bowls and top with a dollop of the yogurt mixture. Sprinkle with the remaining almonds before serving.

Nutritional information per serving: 345 kcals, 26g fat, 16g net carbo-hydrates, 7.6g protein

Hot Chocolate Brownies

As previously mentioned, I was a strict vegetarian for over 25 years. During this time, I also avoided eggs, so I spent quite a bit of time trying to design the perfect cake recipe. This recipe uses oil. You can, of course, use any oil, but I prefer to use coconut oil or olive oil. These brownies can be eaten cold, but they lose their gooeyness when chilled. They are truly delicious hot with a dollop of coconut cream or coconut yogurt.

Makes 9 brownies
   225g spelt, buckwheat or gluten-free flour
   1 tsp baking powder
   120g cacao or unsweetened cocoa powder
   150g xylitol or erythritol, or stevia drops, to taste
   200ml coconut oil, melted, or light olive oil
   1 tsp vanilla bean paste
   50g extra-dark chocolate chips

Preheat the oven to 180°C (160°C fan oven) Gas 4 and line a traybake tin with baking parchment. Sift the flour, baking powder and cacao into a large bowl. Tip in any bran remaining in the sieve.

   Add 350ml water, the sweetener, oil and vanilla bean paste and whisk until thoroughly mixed.

   Add the chocolate chips and mix thoroughly, then pour into the prepared tin. Bake for 25–30 minutes until firm to the touch. Leave to cool in the tin on a wire rack for 5 minutes before cutting into 9 squares. Serve hot or cold.

Nutritional information per serving: 417 kcals, 29g fat, 36g net carbohydrates, 6.6g protein

Creamy Lemon Mousse

This mousse uses soaked cashew nuts to get the creamy texture. You need to soak them for at least one hour beforehand, so plan this dish ahead. I do not add any sweetener to this, as I don't think it needs it, but if you have a sweet tooth you might want to add a little.

Serves 4

   200g cashew nuts
   150ml coconut cream
   zest and juice of 2 lemons
   1 tsp vanilla extract
   1–2 tbsp Sukrin Fibre or rice malt syrup, or a few drops of
       vanilla stevia liquid, to taste (optional)
   lemon zest or raspberries to decorate

Put the cashew nuts in a bowl and pour over water to cover. Leave to soak for 1 hour, then drain in a colander.

   Put the nuts in a food processor. Add the coconut cream, lemon zest and juice, and vanilla extract. Add sweetener, if using. Whizz until smooth.

   Pour into four serving dishes and chill in the fridge for 2 hours or until set. Serve with a sprinkle of lemon zest or a few fresh raspberries to decorate.

Nutritional information per serving 440 kcals, 37g fat, 12g net carbohydrates, 12g protein

Variation: Instead of lemon, you can use strawberries, raspberries or blueberries.

Vegan Strawberry Gelato

Bananas and mangos are a great base for an ice cream, as when frozen and whipped, they are a really smooth and creamy. I freeze bananas once they start to go brown, as my fussy boys won't eat them once they have the slightest brown mark on them! You can also buy all these ingredients already frozen if you prefer.

Serves 10
  2 mangoes, peeled and roughly chopped
  2 bananas, peeled and roughly chopped
  200g fresh or frozen strawberries
  500ml coconut cream or coconut yogurt

Put the mangoes and bananas into a freezer bag and freeze for 2 hours or overnight until solid.

Put the mangoes and bananas into a food processor and add the remaining ingredients, then whizz until smooth and creamy.

Serve immediately. (Alternatively, transfer to a freezer-proof container and re-freeze until needed. Remove from the freezer at least 5 minutes before serving to soften it slightly.)

Nutritional information per serving: 236 kcal, 18g fat, 14g net carbohydrates, 3g protein

Healthy Snacks

We all love to snack; however, we do have to be a bit careful not to continually eat throughout the day, as that can mean that we eat too much. It is far better to eat meals that keep us fuller for longer. If we do snack, it's best to try to ensure it is a healthy snack that is lower in carbohydrates and sugars.

It is important to identify the triggers of snacking, as they may not always be down to hunger. Snacking can be about emotional eating, boredom, or even thirst, as we often confuse hunger with thirst pangs. Mindless eating is another consideration. We often eat our meals or snack in front of the television, and this can lead to us overeating, because we have stopped listening to our fullness signals and become unaware of what we are eating. Years ago, UK hypnotist, Paul McKenna, ran an experiment on conscious eating. He gave cinemagoers some popcorn as they went into the cinema. It was only when they were offered more of the same popcorn as they left the cinema that they realised the popcorn was stale – no one was aware of this when they were eating it during the film.

The following chapter includes some good ideas for healthy savoury and low-sugar snacks. Don't be tempted to fill up on dried fruit, because they are simply comprised of pure sugar, so find another option. I have also listed below some quick-and-easy snack ideas:

- Nut butter (see page 238) spread on vegetables or fruit.
- Vegetable sticks dipped in hummus, guacamole or salsa (see the chapter on Salads and Dips starting on page 131).
- Granola (see page 93).

Kale Crisps

These are really tasty, so do try them. You can coat them with whatever spices you like, ranging from chilli, garlic, or even nutritional yeast flakes, which gives them a cheese flavour. You can keep things quite simple, on the other hand, and opt for sea salt, black pepper and paprika, as it gives a nice simple flavour that is also suitable for children, but the combination below is my personal favourite.

Makes 200g
    1 tbsp coconut oil, melted, or olive oil, plus extra for greasing
    200g kale
    1 tsp paprika
    1 tsp garlic powder
    ½ tsp thyme
    ½ tsp chilli powder
    coarse sea salt and ground black pepper

Preheat the oven to 150°C (130°C fan oven) Gas 2 and grease a baking tray. Wash and dry the kale in a tea towel or using kitchen paper, making sure it is perfectly dry. Remove any stems and thick bits, just leaving the leaves. Cut into equal lengths.

Put in a bowl and add the oil and flavourings. Combining well to ensure it is all evenly coated.

Put onto the prepared baking tray and cook in the oven for 20–30 minutes until dried but not over-browned. Turn off the oven and leave the kale in the oven to help them dry out more. Remove when cool, and enjoy! Store in an airtight container for up to 4–5 days.

Nutritional information per 100g: 107 kcals, 7.2g fat, 0.81g net carbohydrates, 1.4g protein

---

Using a dehydrator

If you find that you are interested in dried foods, you could invest in a dehydrator. I was sent a dehydrator to review, and I can highly recommend them. The kale crisps come out far drier and crisper than when cooked in the oven.

Root Vegetable Crisps

You can use any root vegetable in this recipe, or a mixture, which is a great way to use up any odd pieces you might have. I have used sweet potato, but potatoes, beetroot and parsnips work equally well. The best way to get perfectly thin crisps is to use a mandoline slicer. These are incredibly sharp and can easily slice a finger, so be careful. If you want to vary the flavour, a tablespoon of nutritional yeast flakes will give a hint of cheese while half a teaspoon of chilli flakes will add more spice.

Makes about 500g
  1 tbsp coconut oil, melted or olive oil, plus extra if needed,
    and extra for greasing

2 sweet potatoes
½ tsp onion granules
½ tsp garlic powder
1 tsp paprika
1 tsp dried oregano
salt and ground black pepper

Preheat the oven to 170°C (150°C fan oven) Gas 3 and grease a baking tray. Slice the sweet potatoes using a mandoline to make thin slices.

Put the slices in a bowl and drizzle with the oil. Add the flavourings and ensure that they are evenly distributed over the potato slices.

Put onto the prepared baking tray, ideally without overlapping them. You can sprinkle over more oil once they are on the baking tray, if needed.

Bake for 10–15 minutes until they are crisp and golden. Remove from the oven and put the crisps on a sheet of kitchen paper to help absorb any excess oil. Leave to cool before storing in an airtight container for up to 4–5 days.

Nutritional information per 30g serving: 33 kcals, 0.8g fat, 5.9g net carbohydrates, 0g protein

Spicy Seed Mix

This is not only great as a snack but it can also be delicious as a salad topping or as a savoury crumble. You can make these on a hob, frying them in coconut oil to get the same baked flavour, but I prefer the ease of the oven, and I normally bung these in while the oven is being used for another dish.

Makes about 250g

> 1 heaped tbsp coconut oil, melted, plus extra for greasing
> 250g mixed pumpkin and sunflower seeds
> 1 tbsp soy sauce or coconut aminos
> 1 tsp paprika
> 1 tsp chilli flakes
> salt and ground black pepper

Preheat the oven to 170°C (150°C fan oven) Gas 3 and grease a baking tray. Put the seeds in a bowl, add the oil, soy sauce, paprika and chilli flakes, and combine well. Season to taste with salt and pepper.

Spread the seeds out onto the prepared baking tray and cook in the oven for 5–8 minutes until golden. Allow to cool. Store in an airtight container for up to one week.

Nutritional information per 15g serving: 89 kcals, 7.3g fat, 2.2g net carbohydrates, 3.2g protein

Nutty Trail Mix

This is my take on the traditional trail mix – and it takes only minutes to prepare. Due to the high fructose content of regular trail mix, I have not included any dried fruit. If you want to add a little bite of sweetness, you can add some chocolate chips, although keep the sugar levels down by opting for dark chocolate – at least 85% cocoa content.

Makes about 400g

> 3 tsp coconut oil, melted, plus extra for greasing
> 60g almonds
> 60g Brazil nuts
> 60g macadamia nuts

60g hazelnuts

30g pumpkin seeds

30g sunflower seeds

1 tsp vanilla extract

1 tsp ground cinnamon

30g coconut flakes

40g vegan dark chocolate or cacao chips (at least 85% cocoa
solids) (optional), broken into pieces

Preheat the oven to 170°C (150°C fan oven) Gas 3 and grease a baking tray. Put the nuts and seeds in a bowl.

Mix together the coconut oil, vanilla extract and cinnamon.

Pour this over the nut mixture and combine well, ensuring everything is evenly coated.

Spread out the nut mixture onto the prepared baking tray and bake for 8 minutes or until golden.

Remove from the oven and leave to cool, then add the coconut flakes and chocolate chips, if using. Store in an airtight container for up to 2 weeks.

Nutritional information per 15g serving: 101 kcals, 9.4g fat, 1.3g net carbohydrates, 2.1g protein

Finger-Licking Nuts

These are really moreish, so you have been warned! You can, of course, use any nut or combination of nuts.

Makes about 300g

300g mixed nuts

1–2 tsp chilli powder, to taste

1 tsp garlic powder

1 tsp dried thyme

2 tsp paprika

1 tbsp coconut oil, melted, or olive oil

coarse sea salt and ground black pepper

Preheat the oven to 170°C (150°C fan oven) Gas 3. Put all the ingredients in a bowl and combine well, ensuring the nuts are equally covered.

Spread out onto a baking tray and bake for 8 minutes or until golden. Remove from the oven and allow to cool. Store in an airtight container for up to 2 weeks.

Nutritional information per 30g serving: 197 kcals, 18g fat, 2.3g net carbohydrates, 4.9g protein

Chilli Roasted Almonds

Almonds are great for heart health and are packed with healthy fat, magnesium, vitamin E and fibre. They are really good for you – but be careful not to eat a whole bowlful, as moderation is still key!

Makes About 300g

300g whole almonds

1–2 tsp chilli flakes, to taste

1–2 tsp chilli powder, to taste

1–2 tsp coarse sea salt or Himalayan salt

1 tbsp coconut oil, melted, or olive oil

Preheat the oven to 170°C (150°C fan oven) Gas 3. Put all the ingredients in a bowl and combine well, ensuring all the almonds are equally covered in the oil, chilli and salt.

Spread out onto a baking tray and bake for 8 minutes or until golden. Remove from the oven and allow to cool. Store in an airtight container for up to 2 weeks.

Nutritional information per 100g: 627 kcals, 54g fat, 6.7g net carbohydrates, 18.7g protein

Savoury Cheese-Flavoured Popcorn

I don't eat popcorn, but my family love it. This is a tasty savoury version, to replace the heavily processed kind.

Serves 6
  1 tbsp coconut oil or olive oil
  50g popcorn kernels
  1–2 tbsp nutritional yeast flakes, to taste (depending on
    cheese strength!)
  1 tsp paprika
  ½ tsp onion powder
  ½ tsp garlic powder
  salt and ground black pepper

Melt the oil in a saucepan over a medium heat, then add the popcorn and put on the lid. Increase the heat to high and allow the popcorn to pop for at least 5 minutes – shaking occasionally. The noise will eventually stop, indicating that all the popcorn has popped.

Remove from the heat and add the nutritional yeast flakes, paprika, onion powder and garlic powder. Combine well and season with salt and pepper to taste. Serve immediately. Store in freezer bags or an airtight container for up to 4–5 days.

Nutritional information per 50g serving: 211 kcals, 4g fat, 33g net carbohydrates, 6.9g protein

Sweet treats

This part of the chapter on healthy snacks contains sweet treats, although all of the recommendations are sugar-free and low in fructose. Check the ingredients of your chocolate to make sure it is vegan. I use 100 per cent Montezuma Absolute Black, but I am very used to the intense, rich taste of 100 per cent cocoa. You may want to start on 85 per cent and build up.

Be careful with some of the 'healthy' bars and snacks that you can buy, especially those promoted as free from refined sugar. Don't be fooled: these often have a base of dates or similar dried fruit, and can pack as large a sugary punch as standard confectionary.

Dark Chocolate Acai Coconut Bars

These are really easy to make, and kids love them, especially the vibrant violet colour. They may seem a bit of a hassle to make but they store well in the freezer, so you can batch cook. Acai powder is packed with antioxidants and is great to add to smoothies, desserts or even soups. You can now buy this from most supermarkets. If you can't find it, you can just make these without, more like the traditional Bounty bars.

Makes 8

    200g desiccated coconut

    2 tbsp coconut oil, melted

    1–2 tbsp rice malt syrup or erythritol or xylitol, to taste, or
        stevia drops to taste

    4 tbsp coconut cream

    2 tsp acai powder or blueberry powder

    150g dark chocolate (minimum 85% cocoa solids) or raw
        cacao, broken into pieces

Combine all the ingredients, except for the chocolate, in a bowl.

Mould into 8 sausage shapes and put onto a baking tray. Put the tray in the freezer and leave until frozen.

Melt the chocolate in a heatproof bowl over a pan of gently simmering water, making sure the base of the bowl doesn't touch the water. Remove the coconut bars from the freezer and coat each one with the chocolate: you can dip them into the chocolate or spoon it on to coat one side at a time, turning them once set. Put each one on a sheet of baking parchment once coated. Put the bars in the fridge or freezer until set. Store in the fridge for 4–5 days or freeze them.

Nutritional information per serving: 372 kcals, 35g fat, 6.5g net carbohydrates, 3.4g protein

Berry Fruit Leathers

These are a great on-the-go snack for adults as well as kids, and are far healthier than the processed variety available in the supermarket. Although they do contain natural fructose, opting for berries helps to keep this in check. They are surprisingly simple to make, and are cooked in a very low oven.

Makes about 15 rolls
  300g strawberries or raspberries
  300g blueberries
  juice of 1 lemon
  1–2 drops of liquid stevia, to taste (optional)

Preheat the oven to 140°C (120°C fan oven) Gas 1 and line a baking tray with a silicon mat or baking parchment. Put all the ingredients into a blender and whizz until smooth.

Spread out the mixture on the prepared baking tray until it is completely covered. Bake for 4–5 hours until dry to the touch all over. The idea is to dehydrate the mixture.

Remove from the oven and leave to cool slightly, then cut into strips lengthways 2–3cm wide. You can put baking parchment cut to size onto each strip to prevent the fruit leather from sticking together once rolled up. Roll up. Store in an airtight container for up to 4–5 days.

Nutritional information per roll: 18 kcals, 0g fat, 3.1g net carbohydrates, 0g protein

Chocolate Almond and Goji Berry Bark

Use dark chocolate for this bark, as it contains less sugar. You can sprinkle the chocolate with a variety of nuts, seeds or fruit, so feel free to adapt the recipe to suit your taste or what is in your store-cupboard.

Makes 12 pieces
  200g dark chocolate (at least 80% cocoa solids), broken
    into pieces
  2 tsp coconut oil or olive oil

2 tbsp coconut flakes

2 tbsp goji berries

2 tbsp flaked almonds

Line a baking tray with baking parchment. Melt the chocolate and oil in a heatproof bowl over a pan of gently simmering water, making sure the base of the bowl doesn't touch the water.

Pour onto the prepared baking tray, spreading it evenly with a palate knife. Sprinkle over the remaining ingredients, pushing them down slightly to help secure them into the chocolate.

Put the tray into the fridge for at least 1 hour or until set. Cut into 12 squares. Store in an airtight container in the fridge for up to 4–5 days.

Nutritional information per serving: 168 kcals, 14.9g fat, 4.9g net carbohydrates, 2g protein

Chocolate Nut Truffles

Some of the truffles on sale have a base of dates or cashew nuts, which makes them very sweet and high in fructose. This is a simple, yet delicious recipe using a base of cocoa, chocolate and water! They are rich and very chocolatey. If you would like to sweeten them, you could add some natural sweetener syrup such as Sukrin Fibre or rice malt syrup.

Makes about 28 truffles

    200ml unsweetened almond milk or other plant-based milk

    250g dark, vegan chocolate (at least 85% cocoa solids), broken into pieces

    50g finely chopped nuts (such as hazelnuts, walnuts, Brazil nuts, pecan nuts or almonds)

    60g cacao powder or unsweetened cocoa powder

Put the milk in a small saucepan over a medium-high heat and bring it gently to the boil, without allowing it to boil over.

Remove from the heat and add the chocolate. Use a balloon whisk to beat it until it starts to form a smooth consistency.

Add the chopped nuts and combine well to ensure the nuts are evenly distributed.

Put the bowl into the fridge and leave for 2–3 hours until cool and set.

Put the cacao powder on a plate. Take a heaped teaspoonful of the chocolate mixture and form it into a ball, then roll it in the cacao powder. Cover a baking tray with baking parchment. Put the ball on the prepared baking tray. Repeat with the remaining mixture. Store in an airtight container in the fridge for up to 4–5 days.

Nutritional information per truffle: 77 kcals, 6.4g fat, 2.4g net carbohydrates, 1.7g protein

Variations: You can omit the nuts if you prefer, and add some orange zest and ½ tsp orange essence to create your own chocolate orange truffles. These are also lovely filled with dried raspberries and strawberries.

Sweet Cinnamon Pecan Nuts

These spiced nuts remind me of the flavours of Christmas. They are really nice to have on top of some coconut yogurt or with some chopped dried apple.

Makes about 300g
    300g pecan nuts
    2 tbsp coconut oil, melted
    2 tsp ground cinnamon, plus extra to sprinkle if needed

1 tsp ground allspice

1 tsp ground mixed spice

2 tsp Sukrin Gold (optional)

Preheat the oven to 150°C (130°C fan oven) Gas 2. Put the pecan nuts in a bowl and add the oil, spices and Sukrin Gold, if using.

Combine well, ensuring they are completely covered. Spread out onto a baking tray in a single layer. You can finish with a sprinkle of cinnamon, if you are unsure whether they are evenly coated.

Cook in the oven for 5–8 minutes until golden – no more or they will start to burn. Remove and allow to cool. Store in an airtight container for up to 4–5 days.

Nutritional information per 30g serving: 191 kcals, 16.5g fat, 2.1g net carbohydrates, 5.7g protein

Everyday Basic Recipes

This chapter features the basic recipes referred to in some of the recipes in this book. Some of them are also great to keep in your store-cupboard. You may not have thought about making your own nut butter, but once you see how ridiculously easy it is, as well as exceptionally tasty, you might change your mind.

The emphasis of this book is on optimum health and choosing a food for its nutritional benefits. When we rely on processed foods, our diet lacks vital nutrients. Opting to make the essentials from scratch feeds our body and also our soul. Please take your time to read through these recipes – believe me, you will be surprised at how simple they really are.

Almond Milk

You could be forgiven for thinking that making your own nut milk is a step too far, but I have included my recipe in case you would like to try. It actually takes very little time and it doesn't involve much work – you just leave the nuts to soak overnight and then whizz them in a blender. This recipe uses almonds, but you can use any other nut.

Makes about 1 litre
   120g almonds (or nuts of your choice)
   2 tbsp almond butter

Put the almonds in a bowl and cover with water. Leave overnight then drain in a colander.

Put the nuts into a blender, food processor or Nutribullet. Add 1 litre water and the nut butter, then whizz until smooth.

Strain through a muslin into a jug and pour into a jar. Cover and store in the fridge and use within 5 days.

Nutritional information per 100ml: 85 kcals, 7.2g fat, 1g net carbohydrates, 2.9g protein

Vegan Parmesan

This is really more of a seasoning than a cheese alternative, but it works well to replace Parmesan cheese, not just to top your dishes but also to add to polenta to create a crispy coating. I make this and store it in a jar until needed. It's surprising how a sprinkle can lift a meal.

Makes 200g
   100g walnuts
   75g nutritional yeast flakes
   1 tsp garlic granules
   2 tbsp onion granules
   2 tsp paprika
   salt and ground black pepper

Put the walnuts into a food processor and whizz until they resemble fine crumbs. Pour into a bowl and add the remaining ingredients.

Season with salt and pepper, then stir until thoroughly combined. Transfer to a jar and store for up to 1–2 weeks.

Nutritional information per tablespoon (15g) 81 kcals, 5.9g fat, 1.3g net carbohydrates, 4.6g protein

Nut Butters

You can buy a variety of nut butters, but always check the ingredients, as they can contain palm oils and added ingredients when they should only contain nuts. The flavour of homemade nut butter, however, is fantastic and I love using them in my cooking. This is such a simple recipe, I urge you to give homemade nut butters a go – you might find that you will be converted and ditch the shop-bought varieties.

All nuts are good to use; cashew nuts are higher in carbohydrate than other nuts, whereas macadamia nuts are the highest in fat.

Makes 400g
400g nuts of your choice, such as almonds (Brazil nuts and
macadamia nuts are my favourites)

Preheat the oven to 170°C (150°C fan oven) Gas 3. Put the nuts on a baking tray and roast gently for 8–10 minutes until lightly golden. This will help to release more of the oils and the flavour. Do not let the nuts burn.

Remove from the oven and leave to cool slightly. Transfer to a food processor or Nutribullet and blend: it will first form a dust, but keep going, as it will then start to form a butter. The more you process, the smoother the butter. This can take several minutes, but please keep going, it will finally come together!

Transfer to sterilised jars and put them in the fridge until needed.

Nutritional information per tablespoon (15g portion) of almond butter: 93 kcals, 7.9g fat, 1.1g net carbohydrates, 3.1g protein

Sterilising jars: Wash the jars thoroughly, then put them upturned on a baking sheet and dry them in the oven preheated at 140°C (120°C fan oven) Gas 1 for 10–15 minutes. Alternatively, wash the jars then put them in the dishwasher for the hottest cycle.

Variations: You can combine any nuts to create your own flavours; for example, you can also add chia seeds, cocoa, creamed coconut or salt. You can also flavour with vanilla extract, concentrated espresso, or even salted caramel flavouring. When adding any additional ingredients or flavours, do this after you have blitzed the nuts to form a butter, then blitz again to combine well.

Pesto, Pastes and Sauces

We tend to rely far too much on convenience foods, and it's particularly easy to grab a jar of pasta sauce or pesto, rather than make our own. Hopefully, these quick and easy recipes will help you change that. They can be stored in the fridge or frozen until needed and are a great way of using up any spare vegetables and herbs.

Sun-Dried Tomato and Basil Pesto

This pesto is bursting with great flavours and is perfect for adding to spiralised courgette or to soups, or as a topping for a healthy pizza.

Makes 1 small jar (serves 6)
    125g sun-dried tomatoes
    1 large handful of basil leaves
    75g pine nuts
    3–4 garlic cloves, to taste
    4 tbsp extra virgin olive oil (or the oil from the
        sun-dried tomatoes)
    seasoning to taste

Put all the ingredients into a blender or food processor and whizz until smooth and combined.

Pour into a dish, cover and put in the fridge for at least 30 minutes to allow the flavours to infuse.

Store in the fridge in an airtight container for up to 1 week. You can also freeze it: spoon the pesto into an ice-cube tray and freeze, then pop out a few cubes when you need them.

Nutritional information per serving: 277 kcals, 28g fat, 2g net carbohydrates, 2.7g protein

Chilli and Coriander Pesto

There is no reason why pesto can't have a bit of a kick, and this one certainly delivers. This pesto adds a powerful zing to everyday recipes. I use this with spiralised butternut squash and top it with a few pine nuts and walnuts. A warning: it can be very addictive!

Makes about 250g
    1–2 red chillies, to taste, deseeded
    1 large handful of coriander leaves
    60g baby leaf spinach

75g pine nuts

3–4 garlic cloves, to taste

4 tbsp extra virgin olive oil

seasoning to taste

Put all the ingredients in a food processor or blender and whizz until smooth and combined.

Pour into a dish, cover, and put in the fridge for at least 30 minutes, to allow the flavours to infuse.

Store in the fridge in an airtight container for up to 1 week. You can also freeze it: spoon the pesto into an ice-cube tray and freeze, then pop out a few cubes when you need them.

Nutritional information per 15g serving 61 kcals, 6.1g fat, 0g net carbohydrates, 0g protein

Spicy Harissa Paste

I love spicy food, but find it frustrating when a lot of the pastes contain sugar and poor-quality oils. I use this pasta a lot to add a kick to everyday meals. It is really delicious with some roasted vegetables and rice, or you can add it to your base dish, Moroccan style dishes, chillies – or even in a curry.

■ Get ahead – this dish can be prepared in advance

Makes about 250g

2 tsp coriander seeds

2 tsp cumin seeds

2 tsp caraway seeds

2 tsp mustard seeds

2 star anise
3 red chillies, deseeded
4 garlic cloves, cut in half
1 tbsp paprika
2 tbsp sun-dried tomato paste
4 tbsp olive oil
zest and juice of 1 lemon
seasoning to taste

Put the seeds and star anise into a saucepan and dry-fry for 5 minutes to help release the flavours. Remove the star anise and discard.

Pour the seeds into a food processor or Nutribullet. Add the remaining ingredients and whizz until it forms a smooth paste. You may need to stop halfway through processing and scrape down the side of the processor, and whizz again to ensure it is all combined well.

Store in an airtight container in the fridge for up to 5 days. You can freeze it: spoon the paste into an ice-cube tray and freeze, then pop out a cube when you need it.

Nutritional information per 15g serving: 52kcals, 4.9g fat, 1g net carbohydrates, 0g protein

Red Thai Paste

This is a punchy paste that can add flavour to lots of dishes. Add it to soups or noodles.

Makes 1 small jar
4 tbsp olive oil
3 red chillies, deseeded and finely chopped
4 garlic cloves

½ red onion
3cm piece of fresh ginger, peeled and grated
3 lemongrass stalks, tough outer covering removed
zest and juice of 1 lime
3 tbsp paprika
3 tsp cumin seeds
3 tsp coriander seeds
4 sun-dried tomatoes
a small bunch of coriander leaves

Put all the ingredients into a food processor or Nutribullet and whizz to form a paste. Transfer to a jar and store in the fridge for up to 3 weeks.

Nutritional information per 15g serving: 31 kcals, 2.7g fat, 0.9g net carbohydrates, 0.4g protein

Olive Tapenade

A tapenade is very versatile and is great added to pasta, on roasted vegetables, spread on toast or served as a dip. I have used black olives in this recipe, but you can use green if you like. I like my tapenade to have a touch of chilli heat, but you can omit the chilli if you prefer a milder tapenade.

Makes about 300g
    200g pitted black Kalamata olives
    2 garlic cloves, halved
    1–2 red or green chillies, to taste (optional), deseeded
    1 tbsp capers
    40g whole almonds
    2 tbsp olive oil

    1 tbsp soy sauce or coconut aminos
    zest and juice of ½ lemon
    a small handful of parsley leaves
    salt and ground black pepper

Put all the ingredients, except the salt and pepper, into a food processor or Nutribullet and whizz until it forms a smooth paste. You may need to stop halfway through processing and scrape down the sides of the processor, then whizz again to ensure it is all combined well.

Taste and add seasoning to taste: I love to add lots of black pepper. Store in an airtight container in the fridge for up to 5 days.

Nutritional information per 15g serving: 47kcals, 4.4g fat, 0.8g net carbohydrates, 0.7g protein

Basic Vegetable Stock

I prefer to make my own stock for flavour and to ensure it doesn't contain lots of additives or salt. All stock can be frozen. I pop portions of about 300ml into freezer bags and freeze, ready to add from frozen to my dishes. Any vegetable will go well with the stock, apart from swede, cabbage and broccoli, as these can overpower the stock.

▣ Get ahead – this dish can be prepared in advance

Makes about 1.5 litres
    2 tsp coconut oil or olive oil
    2 onions, roughly chopped
    2–4 garlic cloves, to taste, roughly chopped
    1 leek, chopped
    4 celery sticks, roughly chopped

2 carrots, chopped

2 bay leaves

3 thyme or rosemary sprigs

1 tsp paprika

1 tsp onion granules

salt and ground black pepper

Heat the coconut oil in a large saucepan over a medium heat and cook the onions, garlic, leek, celery and carrots for 5 minutes, stirring continuously.

Add the remaining ingredients, then add 1.5 litres boiling water, or to cover.

Bring to the boil then reduce the heat and simmer for 30 minutes. Alternatively, transfer to a slow cooker and cook on low for 6 hours.

Strain the vegetables through a sieve over a large bowl, pressing the vegetables into the sieve to obtain the most flavour.

Pour into a jug and store in the fridge until needed. You can also pour portions of 300ml stock into freezer bags and freeze.

Basic Tomato Sauce

This is a very versatile sauce. You can use it as a basic tomato sauce to accompany a pasta dish, lasagne or casserole or you can use as a topping for pizza. This is so much nicer than store-bought jars of pasta sauce. It keeps in the fridge for a week and also freezes well.

Makes 2 jars (approx. 1kg)

1 tsp coconut oil or olive oil

1 large red onion, diced

3 garlic cloves, roughly chopped

1 large red pepper, diced

1kg tomatoes, diced
150ml red wine
2 sprigs of fresh thyme or 1 tsp dried thyme
2–3 sprigs of fresh oregano or 1 tsp dried oregano
2 sprigs of rosemary or ½ tsp dried rosemary
4 fresh basil leaves or ½ tsp dried basil
small handful fresh parsley or 1 tsp dried parsley
seasoning to taste

Place the oil in a saucepan and heat on a medium heat. Add the onions, garlic and pepper and cook for 2 minutes to start to soften, then add the tomatoes and red wine. If using dried herbs, add them now.

Bring up to a light simmer and cook gently for 10 minutes, stirring occasionally. Add the fresh herbs, if using, and season to taste.

Cook for another 5 minutes. Remove from heat and allow to cool.

When cooled, freeze or store in the fridge in an airtight container or jar for up to 1 week

Nutritional information per 100g: 28 Kcals, 0.1g fat, 3.6g net carbo-hydrates, 0.6g protein

Variation: You can turn this into an arrabiata sauce by adding 2 chillies (or to taste) to the recipe above. You can also add olives and diced aubergine to make a chunky sauce.

Index